EXPOSED

The Electronic Sickening of America and How to Protect Yourself

Includes Dangers of 5G & Smart Devices

2020 Update

BILL CADWALLADER, MBA, EMRS

*Certified
Electromagnetic Radiation Specialist*

with LOIS CADWALLADER, MA

Stop Dirty Electricity
Las Vegas, Nevada

Exposed: The Electronic Sickening of America

Stop Dirty Electricity
Las Vegas, Nevada
StopDirtyElectricity.com

ISBN-10: 1732365008
ISBN-13: 978-1-7323650-0-1

Library of Congress Control Number: 2018906268

HEA021000: HEALTH & FITNESS / Safety

Printed in the United States of America

DEDICATED TO

The memory of Del and Marguerite Simmons—our first health mentors who made a tremendous difference in our lives and brought us great joy!

Disclaimer of Liability

Stop Dirty Electricity does not claim to diagnose, treat, or cure any medical condition or disease. Stop Dirty Electricity shall not be liable for incidental or consequential damages, lost profits, or revenues to the fullest extent such liability may be disclaimed by law.

Contents

Introduction

There's a hidden danger pulsating in the airways and buzzing behind the walls of millions of American homes, schools, and businesses. Our families, co-workers, even our pets, are exposed to electromagnetic radiation (EMR) almost continually, 24/7.

Few people want to address this topic because they don't know what to do. They are frustrated and overwhelmed by the scattered and conflicting information that's out there. And they fear that they will have to give up their electronic necessities.

I felt that way as well—until I learned that the great news is that you CAN take control of your exposure to harmful electromagnetic radiation and learn how to use your electronic devices more safely.

First, some background: A disturbing correlation has been discovered between electro-pollution and a host of diseases and disorders. These include cancer, neurological diseases, respiratory diseases, behavioral disorders, chronic fatigue, ADHD, insomnia, depression, headaches, muscle/joint pain, chronic inflammation, and many more.

The report *BioInitiative 2012*, which updates the earlier *BioInitiative 2007*, collates research from around the world on the bio-effects and health hazards of electromagnetic fields: from wires (power lines, electrical wiring, appliances, etc.) and wireless technologies (cell and cordless phones, cell towers, WiFi, wireless laptops, wireless routers, baby monitors, surveillance systems, wireless utility meters, etc.). It represents more than 3,800 scientific, peer-reviewed studies done by PhDs and MDs on the potential health effects of prolonged exposure to electromagnetic radiation. And the research continues to grow.

One of the most alarming reports comes from a cancer cluster at a middle school. Up to 24 teachers and staff members at the school were diagnosed with various forms of cancer. Thyroid cancer was 13 times greater than expected; melanoma was almost 10 times greater than expected; uterine cancer was more than nine times the expected amount. To date, up to 49 former students also came down with cancer while in their twenties, even though they spent no more than three years in that school. The worst news of all: six teachers and staff members have died, and six students have died.

Why Isn't Everyone Sounding the Alarm?

We'd all like to blame big industry and the enormous profits associated with electronics for neglecting, minimizing and discrediting this issue. While that may be true, we as consumers are often not willing to forfeit the benefits we enjoy from our electronic devices. Well, the good news is that in most cases, we don't have to.

To put you at ease, I want to say that I am not anti-technology. I use it on a daily basis. I have a smartphone and computer, and use social media. This book is about how to use your electronic devices more safely. It is about how to guard yourself and the people you love against the unintended consequences of the digital age. This book is about solutions.

Read it. Do it. Share it.

Pre-Test

1. About how many mobile connections are there world-wide? (9.42 billion)
2. What percentage of adults in the U.S. owns a cell phone? (95%)

3. What is the average amount of time young people use a cell phone or tablet per day in the U.S? (7 hrs.)
4. What is the average number of times U.S. users touch their cell phones in a day? (2,600; heavy users, 5,000+)

(Nelson, 2016; Winnick & Zolna, 2016; Hacker Noon, 2017; Pew Research Center, 2018; Jacobo, 2019; Turner, 2020)

Interestingly, the mobile device usage does not vary much between demographics. It doesn't seem to matter if users live in the city or country, what their income or education is, or what their racial profile is. Usage spans from sea to shining sea. So, you can see that this is a very big issue, involving nearly the entire population of the United States, and a significant percentage of the population worldwide.

A Word to the Skeptics

Maybe you doubt the seriousness of this topic. You are reading this book because you are my friend. Or because you are curious.

You tell me, "I haven't seen enough evidence to be seriously concerned about this topic." To that, I answer—if you are counting on the news media to represent the research, then you won't be concerned. Be assured that you are unlikely to encounter the evidence that you need to reach a well-informed conclusion. The news media is fed press releases by the industry, and the industry is not likely to report a study that disparages its products. That is why I have spent countless hours reading original, independent research.

You say, "Scientists can't agree on any of this." Well, the truth is, the large majority of scientists who have researched the dangers of electromagnetic radiation do agree. That's why I wrote this book.

And you say, "If it were reeeeeally dangerous, we'd all know about it." Know about it? Kind of like tobacco? And asbestos? And lead? And pesticides? And air pollution?

This book addresses all of these objections and provides resources so that you can do your own digging—if you really want to know.

A Word to the Purists

In the United States, there are a small number of you who do not own a cell phone. You may not own one because you don't want the additional exposure to harmful EMR. Some of you may be highly EMR sensitive—exposure to EMR makes you ill. Others of you have recognized that you had a serious digital addiction and you have intentionally disconnected. You've done your homework and are very smart! Additionally, some of you don't own a cell phone because you don't want to be the reason that the next cell tower is put up. You are very principled.

I admire you. I really do. The wireless portion of this book might not be necessary for you. Although, since you cannot move or disable a cell tower, you will have to know how to protect you and your family from a cell tower threat close to you.

That's all well and good. However, I wrote this book for your family and young children, grandchildren, nephews, and nieces. They grew up with electronics. It is in their cultural DNA. They are NOT going to give up their electronic devices. They need to learn how to use their electronics more safely to minimize their exposure. And your neighbors may have wireless devices and that can affect you as well.

So, don't put this book down just yet. In addition to wireless devices, there are other sources of electromagnetic radiation that are often neglected. These include every wire in your home that you cannot see—in the walls, ceilings, and floors, and also wires and cords you can see, as well as high-voltage power lines outside your home. I hope you can glean additional information to further protect yourself and your family and your pets from the dangers hidden behind every wall in your home.

Additionally, there is the real and growing danger of "second-hand" electromagnetic radiation that is becoming more and more unavoidable as our digital culture leans toward becoming totally wireless.

This book has been written to be accessible to people who have little or no technical background in electronics or physics. The grammar and syntax has been relaxed so it's way easy to read. It has many practical solutions that can be accomplished by just about anyone in one minute, and often without cost.

Start reading and thinking about what actions you will take to lower your exposure to electromagnetic radiation.

Or, if you need or want solutions right now, go to Chapters 7 and 8 (more than 30 pages of solutions) and Appendix I for your Comprehensive Home Safety Audit.

10 WAYS YOU CAN REDUCE

MOVE ALL

❶ Electronic devices, including chargers and clocks, as far away as possible at night to reduce radiation through the air and from the wires.

ALWAYS

❷ Use speaker phone. Your cell phone is constantly trying to connect to a cell tower, increasing radiation.

TURN OFF

❸ WiFi and Bluetooth and turn ON Airplane mode when carrying a cell phone or tablet close to your body and not in use.

TURN ON

❹ Airplane mode with WiFi and Bluetooth OFF when using a device if you don't need an Internet connection* such as reading a downloaded book.

*On Apple products "not connected" still means radiation is ON.

*REMOVE ROUTER**

❺ From bedroom and living areas and turn it OFF when you sleep or when not using WiFi. Routers produce WiFi and continuously create radiation.

* Make sure that critical devices don't go through router.

RADIATION EXPOSURE NOW!

REPLACE ALL

❻ Cordless home phones with corded land line phones. The base radiates like a router even when not in use.

LEAVE

❼ The room when you use a microwave. The farther you move, the less radiation you'll receive. Reduce overall microwave use.

AVOID

❽ Using portable electronic devices on your lap and turn ALL electronics OFF when not in use. Use them in battery mode and not plugged in and charging.

NEVER

❾ Use a Bluetooth wireless ear piece or wireless headphones. They generate radiation even when not on a call or playing music.

WE RECOMMEND THAT

❿ You do not use a baby monitor. If you want use one, it must be measured to determine if it can be placed at a safe distance for both the baby and parents.

BONUS TIP!

➡ Determine if you have a new electric utility "smart meter" with a digital display. Ask your utility company to "opt out" and return to an analog meter.

SECTION I

The Electronic Sickening of America

Chapter 1

Why Should You Care?

We Don't Know What We Don't Know

Electromagnetic radiation has always existed in nature.

Planet Earth itself has electromagnetic fields.

We are bioelectric beings.

Our heart contractions, pineal glands, and brain waves—just to name a few—all have an electrical component.

In fact, we can't move a muscle without an electrical impulse.

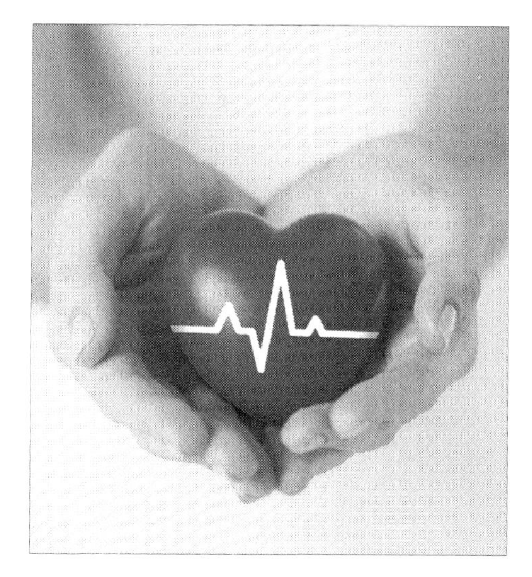

Dr. Gerard J. Hyland told the Global Union Against Radiation Deployment from Space, "The human body is an electrochemical instrument of exquisite sensitivity." (GUARDS, 2015)

He also wrote in a scholarly article published in the prestigious medical journal *The Lancet*, "If mobile phones were a type of food, they simply would not be licensed." (Hyland, 2000)

Dr. Hyland knows whereof he speaks. He is an Honorary Associate Fellow of the University of Warwick, UK, an Executive Member of the International Institute of Biophysics, in Neuss-

Holzheim, Germany, and a Trustee of the UK EM Radiation Trust.

So, what's the difference between electromagnetic radiation in nature and man-made electromagnetic radiation?

Electromagnetic radiation present in nature is a very different kind than what is generated by electromagnetic frequencies (EMF) used in modern technology. To keep it simple, let's compare just five characteristics:

EMFs in Nature	Man-made EMFs
Direct Current	Alternating and Direct Current
Very low frequencies	Much higher frequencies
Very low power density (except lightning)	Much higher power density
Non-polarized	Polarized
Few sources	Huge number of growing sources

Humans have never before been exposed to this type of electromagnetic radiation for long periods of time the way we are during our lifetimes. The continual pulsing and non-pulsing of man-made electromagnetic frequencies and its subsequent electromagnetic radiation has been unleashed and it is almost everywhere, layer upon layer. This is something new. It is foreign to what we find in the natural world. We don't really know how this is all going to turn out. (Levitt, 2007; Firstenberg, 2017)

Why should you care? Your health is at risk.

Here's why I care: I've worked in Information Technology all my life. At one point, I had a co-worker who had his cell phone up to his ear every time I saw him—before meetings, after meetings, sitting at his desk, walking to his vehicle.

He developed a huge tumor at the exact place he positioned his cell phone. He had the tumor surgically removed and was treated with massive amounts of chemotherapy. Even so, the tumor grew back.

He had additional chemo.

Then he died, leaving a wife who is now a widow and seven children who are now fatherless.

At that moment I knew there was something very unsafe about the way we were using our cell phones and other electronic devices, and that the telecommunications industry was not telling us how to use these devices in the safest possible way.

This was the beginning of my search to discover not only the radiation hazards of cell phones, but all electronic devices and electrical wiring. And, most important of all, the solutions on how to use them in a safer way.

I became a Certified Electromagnetic Radiation Specialist. Never heard of one? It's because there are currently only about 30 of us practicing in the United States. We have gone through the rigorous certification process, which takes nearly two years to complete through the Building Biology Institute, and includes ongoing professional development with colleagues and coaches (more info at: hbelc.org).

Think for a minute of all the things we once thought were "safe," that in fact were actually very dangerous:

- Asbestos
- BPA plastics
- Formaldehyde
- Lead in paints and gasoline
- Pesticides
- Tobacco and smoking

And how many years did it take to expose the dangers of these things, reign in the industries promoting these hazardous materials, and educate the people? (See Chapter 3 for the depressing details.)

And now we add:

- Electromagnetic Radiation, or EMR, which is produced by an electromagnetic field or EMF

Electromagnetic radiation is the tobacco of the Digital Age. And, like tobacco and smoking, it can kill you.

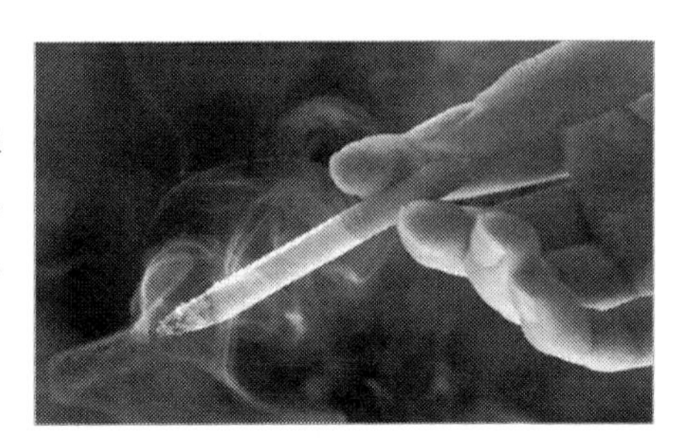

How Much Is Too Much?

According to Olle Johansson, PhD, associate professor in neuroscience at the Karolinska Institute in Sweden, our bodies are subjected to one quintillion times (that's a 1 with 18 zeros behind it) more electromagnetic radiation today than we were a decade ago. In 2017, he was featured in a documentary, *Generation Zapped*, to explain the risks we face.

We are talking about man-made, non-ionizing radiation; i.e., the radiation emitted from cell phone towers, WiFi, smart meters, etc. Regardless of the exact number, it is a very big number. And our exposure is almost constant and grows every year.

Some remember when all we had in the kitchen was a coffee maker, and maybe a toaster. And each room had only one or two electrical outlets. Now, how many electronic devices, wired and wireless, are in our homes? And, like storage, you can never have too many electrical outlets, right? How many electronic devices and outlets can you spot right now? They have become part of our home-scapes.

Now, if you really want an eye-opener, go to: AntennaSearch.com. Type in your address and find out how many cell towers and antennas are within two miles. Unless you live in a rural area, it is usually in the hundreds. Aren't we lucky to have such good reception?

Maybe not.

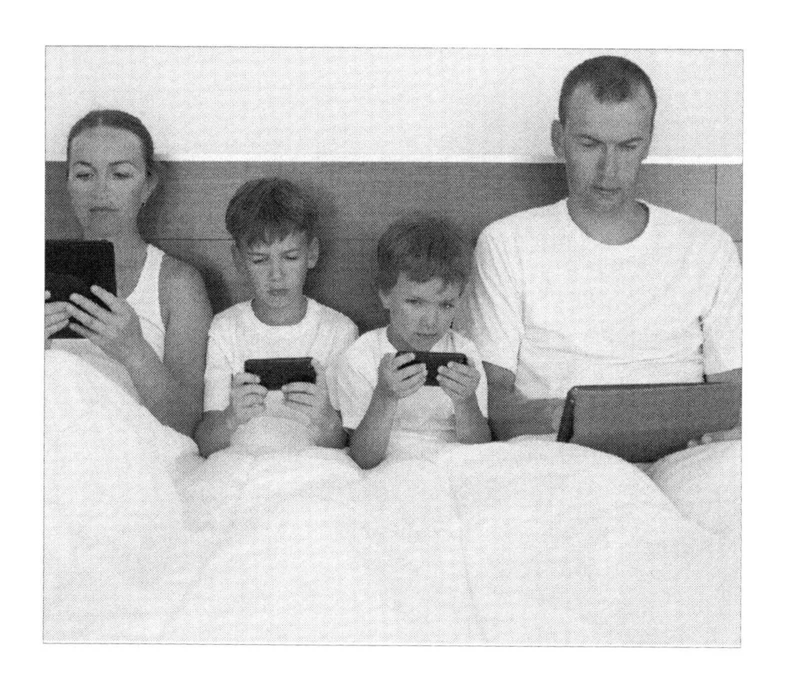

Many published studies confirm the carcinogenicity of electromagnetic radiation, but most studies focus on the biological exposure of only a single frequency. Few published scientific studies as of yet have explored the aggregate biological effects of the complex, multi-frequency radiation that now pollutes modern buildings and the general environment everywhere across the globe. (Wi-Cancer.info)

A 2016 study of the man-made wave pollution within the Stockholm Central Railway Station in Sweden found twenty different pulsed frequency sets. Research was conducted by the Hardell Cancer Research Group. This study is a reality check on the astronomical number of wireless signals that simultaneously bombard our bodies everywhere we go. (Hardell et al., 2016)

For a startling audio-visual representation of this mesh of radiation in which we live, check out the short, 5-minute video,

"She Looks Safe": tinyurl.com/ExposedSheLooksSafe. You might have to advance the home page banner to find it. And be sure to turn up your volume and watch till the end. Prepare to be alarmed.

If we could listen in on these invisible strata surrounding us, what would we hear?

Ping-Ping-Ping
Click-click-click-click
Click-ck-ck-ck-ck-ck-ck-ck
Zapzapzapzapzapzapzapzapzap
Ningngngngngngngngngngngngngng
Shshshshshshshshsshshshshsshshshsshs
Hummmmmmmmmmmmmmmmmmmmmmmmm
Buzzzzzzzzzzzzzzzzzzzzzzzzzzzzzzzzzzzzzzzzzzzzzzzz

Do No Harm

BioInitiative 2019 lists more than 3,800 scientific, peer-reviewed studies on the health hazards of electromagnetic radiation. This research was done by MDs and PhDs from all over the world. And the research is growing every year. (See Appendix II: Resources for Advanced Reading.)

Martin Blank, PhD, reported: "Cells in the body react to EMFs as potentially harmful, just like to other environmental toxins, including heavy metals and toxic chemicals. The DNA in living cells recognizes electromagnetic fields at very low levels of exposure and produces a biochemical stress response. The scientific evidence tells us that our safety standards are inadequate, and that we must protect ourselves from exposure to EMFs due to power lines, cell phones and the like, or risk the known consequences. *The science is very strong and we should sit up and pay attention.*" (emphasis added)

Blank served as a Special Lecturer in the Department of Physiology and Cellular Biophysics at Columbia University's College of Physicians and Surgeons. He conducted research in the field of Bioelectromagnetics and authored the BioInitiative report's section on Stress Proteins.

Researcher Dr. George Carlo warns: "Some of the claims that were being made about health effects were so severe that had there been pre-market testing, cell phones never would have made it into the market place." (Carlo, 2001)

What comes to your mind when you hear the word, RADIATION?

- Images (Rolling Pastures or Industrial Complex?)
- Feelings (Peaceful or Stressful?)
- Colors (Green or Red?)

Instinctively, I think we all now know that radiation is harmful. We innately would not choose to place our pillows under a cell phone tower and expect to sleep in heavenly peace.

We know this about radiation:

1. ***Damages DNA***—that can't be good.

   An increase in DNA strand breaks was observed after exposure to electromagnetic radiation. Researchers speculate that these effects could result from a direct effect of electromagnetic radiation on DNA molecules and/or impairment of DNA-damage repair mechanisms in cells. Subsequent studies further support the results of earlier studies showing the effects of radio frequency electromagnetic radiation on DNA. (Lai, 1996; Lai, 2012; Mihai et al., 2014)

2. ***Compromises the blood-brain barrier***—the permeability of the blood-brain barrier is increased resulting in dangerous chemicals that were never intended to enter the brain now having access.

   The blood-brain barrier is a critical structure in the brain designed to separate the flow of blood through the brain from the brain matter itself. Blood contains toxins, heavy metals, and pathogens being carried to excretory organs and also certain molecules, such as albumin, that can be lethal to brain tissue. A study from Sweden reports that exposure to cell phone radio frequency induces pathological leakage of albumin across the blood-brain barrier.

What stands out in this research is that it took extremely low frequency levels (ELFs) of radiation and as little time as two hours to result in leakage in the blood-brain barrier, which can cause nerve cell damage and neuron death. Yes, it's true that humans have millions of neurons, so the harmful effects may not be immediate. However, the evidence suggests that, as with smoking and other toxins, there is a cumulative effect over time. Do millions of people have to suffer before anything is done to protect us? (IEEE, 2004; Eberhardt et al., 2008; Salford et al., 2012)

Another study reports that this leakage is not just superficial; it was found to be present several centimeters deep in central cerebral structures, including the cortex, hippocampus, and midbrain. (Lin & Lin, 1982)

(The word "leaky" is not a word you would like to be applied to your brain.)

3. ***Weakens the immune system***—and that's on top of all the other assaults upon our health.

During the past decade considerable evidence has accumulated demonstrating that exposure to extremely low-frequency electromagnetic fields (ELFs) can

- Elicit cellular changes.
- Disturb the immune system through various allergic and inflammatory responses.
- Damage tissue repair mechanisms.
- Result in stress protein response.

This assault on the immune system increases the risks for various diseases, including cancer. These and the EMR/EMF effects on other biological processes (e.g., DNA damage, neurological effects, the proliferation of stress proteins, the disruption of cell integrity, and communication, etc.) are now widely reported to occur

Could this be the straw that breaks the camel's back?

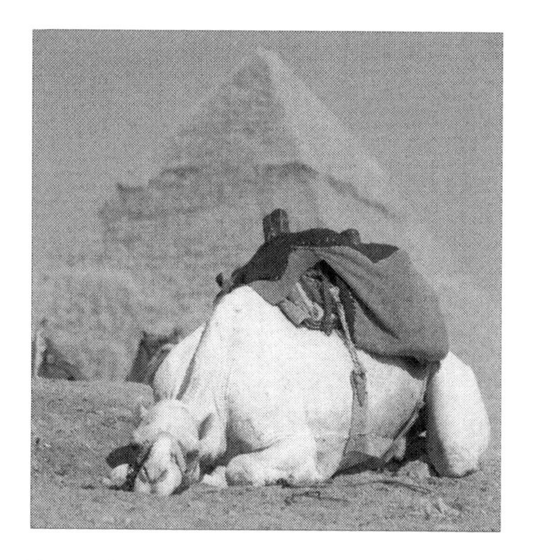

at exposure levels significantly below most current national and international safety limits.

BioInitiative 2019 concludes that the existing public safety limits are inadequate to protect public health, and that new public safety limits are warranted. This is backed up by a number of studies that examined the effects of electromagnetic fields on living cells. (Walleczek, 1992; Johansson, 2009; Blank & Goodman, 2009)

What is this doing to our bodies' natural defenses?

"It is possible that a subset of the population, which may have a genetic predisposition to the development of certain diseases, or who have been exposed to chemical or physical initiating agents, may experience enhanced sensitivity to the promotional effects of electromagnetic fields," states Charles M. Keen in his article, "Possible Biological Effects of Electromagnetic Fields Associated with Electric Power Systems: History and Status of the Issue," published by EMF Services, LLC.

Keen has been professionally involved in EMF-related activities since 1992. His background prior to that time spanned nearly two decades in the telecommunications industry, at a range of technical, engineering, and management positions, including development of test procedures for EMR/EMF communications systems. He is an IAEI certified electrical inspector, a member of the International Association of Electrical Inspectors, and holds a BS degree from the University of Maryland.

Is There Any Part of Your Body You Don't Care About?

My wife recently attended a memorial service for a former student of hers. Twenty-two years old. Testicular cancer. An only son. I wonder, where did he carry his cell phone?

Diseases with Strong Correlation to Excessive EMR Exposure

We are not suggesting that EMRs are the sole cause of the following diseases, but that EMRs could be a significant contributing factor. There is an abundance of evidence supporting strong EMR correlation between exposure levels and various diseases.

For those of us who are middle-aged and above, we can think back to when we were in school and ask, how many people did we know who had cancer? Almost no one. Again, there are a multiplicity of causes of diseases. And maybe we are more aware of cancer now. But the research suggests that radiation is a significant factor, as our exposure today is nearly constant, nearly constant, nearly constant.

As you read this list, think about:

- How many people do you know that HAVE the disease?
- Where do people HOLD their smartphones, laptops, or tablets when using them?
- Where do people generally charge cell phones at NIGHT?
- Where do people CARRY electronic devices?
- And how much TIME do people use electronics close to their bodies?
- And, is there any part of your BODY you do not care about?

Electro-pollution is linked to the following symptoms and conditions:

In the neck and head area: brain tumors, salivary gland cancer, thyroid cancer, acoustic neuroma, cancer of the larynx, esophageal cancer, headaches, persistent nosebleeds, dizziness, tinnitus, cognitive impairment.

In the chest, abdominal, and pelvic areas: breast cancer, stomach cancer, colon cancer, ovarian cancer, uterine cancer, testicular cancer, pancreatic cancer, pancreatitis, kidney cancer, nausea, fertility and reproductive issues.

Cancer of the blood: leukemia, multiple myeloma.

Skin cancer and skin disease: Melanoma, itching and burning of skin, rashes.

Other Disorders: ADD/ADHD, autism, neurological diseases, inflammatory diseases, respiratory diseases, tremors and muscle spasms, weakened immunity, lymphoma, insomnia, chronic fatigue, fibromyalgia, heart palpitations, some types of diabetes, hair loss.

This list is by no means comprehensive.

When you consider the bodily burdens of the air we breathe, the water we drink, the nutritionally compromised food we eat, the chemicals we put on our bodies, and the unusual stress factors of our contemporary culture, the addition of the invisible and inaudible yet ubiquitous "ping-ping-pings" to which we are exposed 24/7 is formidable.

Electromagnetic radiation doesn't just "add" to our environmental toxic load. It multiplies it with layer upon layer of increasing, constant exposure. The links of various diseases to EMR/EMF is strong and the evidence is compelling.

Dr. Neil Cherry measured cancer rates in people living in the vicinity of high-powered radio/TV broadcast towers and produced consistent significant dose relationships. He also compared 40 studies of other diseases, similar to the ones listed above. His research included DNA strand breakage, chromosome aberrations, increased pre-tumor activity in cells, reduced melatonin, altered brain activity, altered blood pressure, and increased brain cancer. (Cherry, 2001; Havas, 2006; Barsam et al., 2012; Plourde, & Plourde, 2016)

The research is voluminous. It is sprinkled throughout this book. There are resources for matching specific conditions with relevant research, so in this book I won't attempt to address every disease associated with EMR. Suggestions for advanced reading are included in Appendix II.

But the good news is: THERE ARE SOLUTIONS. (See Section II.)

I'm not going to tell you to get rid of all your electronics. We all use them. They are not going away. But there are good, better, and best solutions. We can often reduce exposure in a single-family detached home by over 90 percent. Stay tuned.

Text Neck

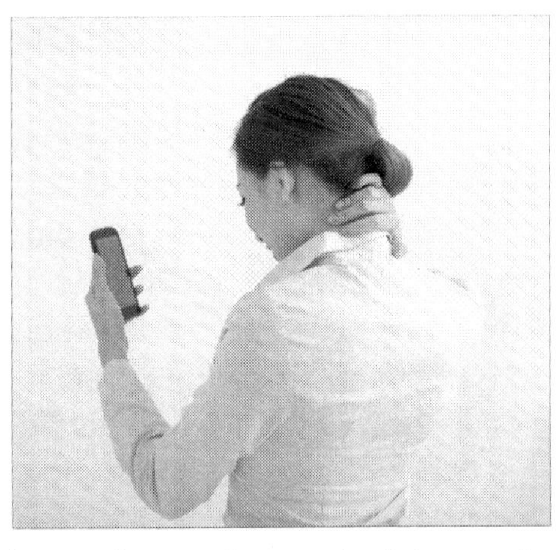

"Text Neck"—try saying that quickly 10 times.

Several years ago, I was walking out of my chiropractor's office, checking my cell phone. He stopped me. He told me to hold the phone UP. That made sense, as I had often heard that the head is like a bowling ball. Now, it seems that the tilt of the head involved in reading and texting is causing serious spinal issues in young people. Next time you are at a concert or sporting event, or even stopped at a stop light, look around and notice how many people are posturing down toward their phones, leaning, slouching, bowing.

An adult head weighs 10-12 pounds in the neutral position. But watch what happens as the head tilts forward, as is the case when looking at a phone and/or texting, according to Kenneth

Hansraj, MD, Chief of Spine Surgery, New York Spine Surgery & Rehabilitation Medicine. At 15 degrees, the force on the neck surges to 27 pounds of pressure.

"Text Neck!" I don't even want to say it, much less endure it. And if you're looking for a career, you might want to consider physical therapy or chiropractic.

Other Digital Injuries

Brian Najarian, MD, a hand surgeon at Cape Cod Orthopedics, treats patients with injuries caused by digital devices. He states that overuse of any body part can cause problems, and hands and fingers are no exception. One of the most common injuries that develops from overuse of the hands is carpal tunnel syndrome. It is a peripheral nerve entrapment that is basically a pinched nerve.

A similar problem that can happen to elbows is called cubital nerve syndrome, commonly called "cell phone elbow."

Painful tendonitis is also reported with excessive use of technology. Dr. John Fatti, founder of the Syracuse Orthopedic Specialists Hand and Wrist Center, says, "We have names for it now—video thumb, smartphone carpal tunnel. People that use their hands in a repetitive, quick way are using the tendons in their hands much more rapidly and much more in an overuse-type situation."

Samsung actually has a disclaimer in its user's guide: "Reduce risk of repetitive motion injuries. When you repetitively perform actions, such as pressing keys, drawing characters on a touch screen with your fingers, or playing games, you may experience occasional discomfort in your hands, neck, shoulders, or other parts of your body. When using your device for extended periods, hold the device with a relaxed grip, press the keys lightly, and take frequent breaks. If you continue to have discomfort during or after such use, stop use and see a physician."

Apple makes this recommendation in its user guide: "When you perform repetitive activities such as typing or playing games on the iPhone, you may experience occasional discomfort in your hands, arms, wrists, shoulders, neck, or other parts of your body. If you experience discomfort, stop using the iPhone and consult a physician."

And then there is the Accidental Texter.

Count out loud:

one thousand one
one thousand two

That's the number of seconds that experts say a driver could safely take his or her eyes off the road.

Now compare that with the number of seconds, on average, drivers actually take their eyes off the road to send text messages. Read it out loud for the greatest impact:

one thousand one
one thousand two
one thousand three
one thousand four
one thousand five
IMPACT!

We've all seen heart-breaking videos about the dangers of texting and driving. Now we call it "Distracted Driving." A lot can happen in five seconds. (Schumaker, 2015)

And as if there were not already enough distractions, there are now Smart Glasses that will notify your retina—yes, your retina—when you have an incoming message. What will this do to the driver who is already distracted? (Chamberlin, 2014)

Check out this awesome seven-minute video: "Intel's New Smart Glasses Hands On": tinyurl.com/ExposedGlasses.

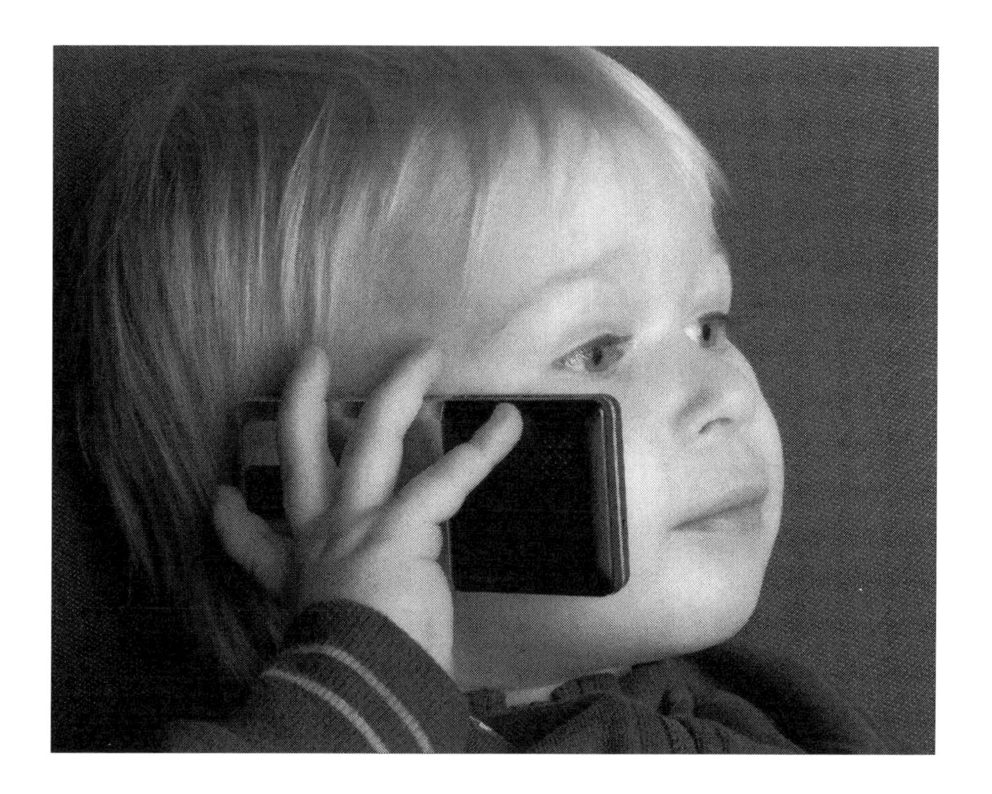

What's It Doing to Our Children?

A paper published online in the journal *Electromagnetic Biology and Medicine* demonstrates that children and small adults absorb significantly more cell phone radiation than had been previously understood by using the conventional "safety guidelines" established in 1996.

If you think about it, it's easy to imagine the relative depth of penetration of a cell phone signal into a child's head, compared to the head of an adult. Let's assume that the EMR "reach" is more than two inches into the cranium. For an adult, whose skull is thicker and whose brain is larger, this might still represent a surface intrusion. But for a small child, this constitutes an assault that is deep into the developing brain.

Dr. Om Gandhi, of the University of Utah, shows how radiation penetrates the skull of an adult (25%), ten-year-old

(50%) and a five-year-old (75%). The younger the child, the deeper the penetration due to the fact that a child's skull is thinner and still developing. Bone marrow in a child's skull absorbs 10 times more microwave radiation than does an adult. (Consumers For Safe Phones, 2011)

A child's brain is still developing and considerbly smaller than that used in the "safety testing model, SAM." It is estimated that twice the radiation than was previously claimed is being absorbed into the head of a child. And what about the baby in the mother's womb? (Gandhi et al., 2012) (See SAR and SAM, Chapter 3.)

Autism: Although the exact cause(s) of autism are hotly debated, one thing upon which we can all agree is that it is becoming more prevalent. Sadly, the autism spectrum is growing. (Doheny, retrieved 2017)

The blame has been pointed to a variety of causes, including genetics, food additives, chemicals and heavy metals, and vaccines. Rarely do the "experts" consider electromagnetic sensitivity, although more and more research is connecting the dots in that direction.

Could ALL of these potential factors be related to EMR/EMF causing a breach in the blood-brain barrier and allowing toxins to intrude the brain? Some experts are suggesting that exposure to EMR/EMF is the potentiating element that allows other offending causes to wreak havoc in the autistic child's brain.

In 2007, Tamara Mariea and George Carlo conducted a study to assess the role of EMF from wireless devices in the cause of autism. The findings of this study suggest a significant role of EMR/EMF in both the cause and the impeded efficacy of therapeutic interventions.

Researchers found that EMR/EMF (specifically from wire-ess devices) trap heavy metals in cells, causing heavy-metal toxicity. This accelerates the onset of autistic symptoms and also impedes therapeutic clearance of the metals. The findings also suggest that EMR/EMF probably work in conjunction with

Identified Prevalence of Autism Spectrum Disorder
ADDM Network 2000 – 2012
Combing Data from All Sites

Surveillance Year	Birth Year	Number of ADDM Sites Reporting	Prevalence per 1,000 Children (Range)	This is about 1 in X children...
2000	1992	6	6.7 (4.5 - 9.9)	1 in 150
2002	1994	14	6.6 (3.3 - 10.6)	1 in 150
2004	1996	8	8.0 (4.6 - 9.8)	1 in 125
2006	1998	11	9.0 (4.2 - 12.1)	1 in 110
2008	2000	14	11.3 (4.8 - 21.2)	1 in 88
2010	2002	11	14.7 (5.7 - 21.9)	1 in 68
2012	2004	11	14.6 (8.2 - 24.6)	1 in 68

other environmental factors (such as chemicals and vaccines) and genetic factors to cause autism. (Mariea & Carlo, 2007)

A separate study was conducted by Dietrich Klinghardt, MD, PhD, and director of the Klinghardt Academy of Neurobiology in Seattle. The researchers measured the mothers' body voltage and microwave exposure in their sleeping environments, and also those of their autistic children. The study strongly suggests that electromagnetic radiation in the sleeping area of the mother during pregnancy, as well as in the sleeping environment of the children, are correlative, if not causal, factors in autism. (Mercola, 2017; Mariea, 2007; Han et al., 2012; Tang et al., 2015; Thornton, 2006)

And with WiFi, wireless, Bluetooth, and smart devices on the rise, could this contribute to the disruption of the protective nature of the blood-brain barrier? In my opinion, the research is robust and should be taken very seriously.

A grandmother's story:

> *One night two years ago, I picked up the phone and listened to my daughter-in-law reveal, "Little Jason has just been diagnosed with autism." We both paused. Then she added that it is a high-functioning Autism.*

As I replay this, I sadly remember that for years, when Jason was a baby, his mom used a baby monitor with strong enough WiFi to send a signal from Jason's crib in his bedroom on one side of the house to upstairs and to the far side of their big Texas home. Jason had that baby monitor close to his body every night and every nap for two years.

And when Jason was a toddler, his techy dad was so pleased to teach him how to hold a smartphone and play challenging games for hours and hours.

Now, at age 6, Jason has been diagnosed with Autism.

What is the cause behind Autism? Genetics? Chemicals? Environment? A combination thereof? I don't think anyone can say for sure. But it certainly does raise questions and give room for caution. I think we can all agree that our children deserve the most caution we can possibly give them.

Childhood leukemia: Are some children wired for this disease? Dr. Nancy Wertheimer did the pioneering study on the effect of electrical wiring configurations and childhood cancer.

An excess of high-voltage electrical wires was noted in Colorado in 1976-1977 near the homes of children who developed cancer, as compared to the homes of control children. The finding was strongest for children who had spent their entire lives at the same address, and it appeared to be dose-related. It did not seem to be associated with neighborhood, street traffic, socio-economic class, or family structure. At that time, it was thought that the source of radiation was from electrical currents traveling on the water pipes or AC magnetic fields. (Wertheimer & Leeper, 1979)

Subsequent studies have confirmed that there is enough epidemiological evidence to show an increased incidence of leukemia in relation to electrical wiring problems creating electromagnetic fields. (Calvente et al., 2010; Milham, 2012; Kundi, 2012)

And now we have cell phones.

Should there be an age requirement on cell phones?

Sir William Stewart, chief science advisor to the United Kingdom from 1990 to 1995 chaired the panel that wrote the influential report "Mobile Phones and Health" in 2000. This report basically said not to worry, just be careful, and watch out for the children.

He subsequently concluded in 2005 that cell phones should not be used by children and that we do not have adequate safety information. "Simple common sense has convinced us that even the remotest possibility of our product becoming a health risk to any child is unacceptable." (BBC News, 2005)

In 2008, a Swedish study concluded that young people may suffer an "epidemic" of brain cancer in later life, and the European Parliament voted 522 to 16 to urge European leaders to develop stricter limits for exposure to radiation from mobile and cordless phones, WiFi, and other devices, partly because children are especially vulnerable. (Lean, 2008)

And in 2012 the Austrian Medical Society issued cell phone safety guidelines stating that cell phones should be used as short a time as possible and that children under 16 should not use cell phones at all.

Try that out on your 14-year-old.

"An ADDICT?" — Not MY Child

In determining what constitutes an addiction, psychologists typically consider frequency of use, amount of money spent, and the degree to which the use interferes with family, social, school, and work relationships.

Additionally, recent brain research demonstrates by way of brain scans, that digital addiction actually changes the way the brain looks and operates. (Kardaras, 2016; Huddleston, 2016)

This is a medical reality. We've never been this way before.

A 2012 article in *Psychology Today* notes that dopamine makes you addicted to seeking information in an endless loop. Interestingly, it is short "bits," such as texts and tweets, that heighten the dopamine response. Dopamine starts you searching, then you get rewarded for the hunt, which makes you search more. Search and find. Search and find. Ding. Dong. Peep. Pop. Cheep. Chirp. BINGO!

It becomes harder and harder to stop looking at email, stop texting, or stop checking your smartphone, or stop playing a video game. I live in Las Vegas. Almost sounds like a slot machine. In fact, author and researcher Brad Huddleston suggests that the Variable Ratio Reward System (where a response is reinforced after an unpredictable number of responses) is a carefully designed, highly addictive formula that is embedded in the most popular and seemingly benign video games. So, as a child mines down into the deeper, intentionally crafted levels of an electronic game, the prompts and responses become more and more addicting. (Huddleston, 2016; Weinschenk, 2012)

Research shows that the effects of these radiation-emitting, highly addictive devices are in fact similar to those provoked by prescription and illegal drugs. (Paz de la Puente & Balmori, 2007)

Do you notice your children feeling a continual leaning toward their phones and tablets? An obsession to connect with phones is rampant, especially among the youth of our society.

Our fingers:

click, swipe,
scroll, tap,
pull, draw,
slip, slide
—all day long!

A research firm, which specializes in consumer reactions to products, recruited 94 Android device users and installed special software on their smartphones. The tool tracked each user's "interaction" all day over a period of five days. As you may recall from the opening pages of this book, the average user touches his or her phone more than 2,600 times a day, according to one study. And heavy cell phone users are said to touch their phones over 5,400 times a day. Where would your children fit in to this range? (Winnick & Robert, 2016)

Electronic Screen Syndrome:

Victoria L. Dunckley, MD, reports the disturbing correlation between electronic screen time and the rise of behavioral disorders in young children in the 2017 article "Electronic Screen Syndrome: An Unrecognized Disorder?" Children's brains are much more sensitive to the use of electronics than we may realize. Research has linked excessive screen time to school problems, aggression, and other behavioral issues. The "sensory overload" causes kids to be overstimulated and "revved up," and they may have a difficult time sleeping, concentrating, or managing stress and regulating their mood.

One study, reported by the Association of American Pediatrics, measured the effects of excessive screen time on children's psychological well-being. The results concluded that children who spent more than two hours per day in front of a screen had greater psychological difficulties, irrespective of physical activity. But it is also estimated that most children far exceed two hours of screen time per day. (Kowalski, 2016)

Isn't it interesting that techno-giants Steve Jobs and Bill Gates both set limitations and boundaries for their children regarding their use of technology. Jobs admitted in a 2011 *New York Times* interview that he prohibited his kids from using the then newly released iPad. Gates told the UK *Mirror* that he and his wife Melinda prohibited their children from owning a cell phone before they turned 14, and their devices were not allowed at dinner time. (Weller, 2018; Stillman, 2017)

And with the advent of "smart schools," our children have additional, almost continual, WiFi exposure while at school. Screen time is now largely a "given" part of the educational process. My wife, a professional educator, observes a dramatic and disappointing decline in the ability of children to follow a sustained, logical, sequential, linear thought. Linear thinking and sequential communication has been replaced by bits and flashes of information, often skipping from topic to topic. Toggle-toggle, flit-flit.

Web psychologist, Liraz Margalit, PhD, compares what is required of a child's brain when listening to a story (processing voice into words, visualizing characters, scenes, and actions, and following a story line, etc.) with a tech-story that spoon-feeds words and images simultaneously, bypassing many important processes whereby a child's developing brain is exercised in cognitive development, language, and imagination. (Margalit, 2016)

Dr. Olle Johansson, Associate Professor and Assistant Professor in Neuroscience, Karolinska Institute, Stockholm, wrote a daring and frank opinion piece questioning the educational value and efficacy of digital learning. (See Appendix IV: "KI-researcher: kick out politicians who give students hazardous e-readers with unproven educational value")

The "Gamification of Education" seems to be the trendiest fad. It's a brilliant marketing stunt to keep up with the epidemic of ADD/ADHD. But is it really working? Or is it actually exacerbating the inability of our children to achieve sustained focus.

What is this doing to our children? How many of these symptoms describe your children or grandchildren, or the children in your neighborhood?

- Irritable
- Depressed
- Excessive tantrums
- Mood swings
- Low frustration tolerance
- Defiant and demanding
- Trouble sleeping
- Disorganized behavior
- Learning difficulties
- Poor short-term memory

(Lai, 2007; Dokoupil, 2012; Davis, 2013; Townsend, 2016)

Perhaps the best way to tell if one is addicted to the phone or not is to watch what happens when it is taken away, or it's out of service. It is, most often, not a pretty sight. There are apps that track your usage and help set time limits.

In all seriousness, digital addiction may require a professional detox program. South Korea is the most "plugged in" country in the world and also has the highest rate of Internet addiction among children in the world. About 200 Digital Detox Retreats, Boot Camps, and treatment centers have sprung up to meet the needs of children and teens who spend every waking moment obsessed with their wireless devices. China has about 300 such centers. (PBS, 2010; Carney, 2015; Chen, 2015)

Children may not be 100 percent of our population, but they are 100 percent of our future!

Example: One day recently my wife and I dined at one of our favorite restaurants off the Las Vegas strip. Shortly after we sat down, a four-year-old boy strode in with his parents and sat at the table next to us. The child was "playing" on his smartphone before the meal was served. He refused to put his phone down, even after the food arrived.

His mother ended up feeding him while he continued to attend to his phone. He never even looked at his food, or his mother. He was transfixed upon the holy glow and intermittently opened his mouth, similar to a baby bird. This continued over the course of the entire meal. While I was horrified at the radiation being inches from this boy's head, my wife was appalled at the obvious parental malfunction. Bon appetit.

Who is guarding our children's physical, mental, and emotional well-being from the collateral damage of our digital culture?

They've Got Us Covered

Have you ever had the feeling that "someone is listening"? Well, they are. And it's more than just your cell phone. Most newer electronic devices are seeded with sensors.

In his 2017 book, *Owned: Property, Privacy and the New Digital Serfdom*, Joshua Fairfield discusses what it means that our environment is seeded with more sensors than ever before. Our computers, dishwashers, smart televisions, Internet-enabled home hubs, smart meters, fitness trackers, and smartphones, just to name a few, constantly gather information about us and our environment. Do we ever take the time to read the license agreement? You might be surprised that our personal information, which is gathered by our smart devices is owned. But not by us. And we agreed to it when we purchased our smart stuff.

I heard on the radio that a fitness tracker company just released its global statistics for the year, proud about tracking the habits of exercise and sleep worldwide. Are you tracked? Probably.

What exactly does that mean? It means at least three things. Smart devices:

- Listen
- Locate
- Log

They Listen

I recently had my own experience with this. I carry my phone on airplane mode with Bluetooth and WiFi off to safeguard against exposure to electromagnetic radiation.

I turned my phone back on to check for messages and saw a friend zipping along on a bike path. "Diane Day! Diane Day," I called out loudly. Well, she was riding so fast that she didn't hear me. But someone else did.

Within a few hours, I had a personal message from her on Facebook . . . but it was suspicious. It didn't sound like her. Sure enough, it was a hacker. Coincidental? Maybe. But the timing is just too close. I can't help but wonder if my phone picked up her name, associated her with my Facebook friend, and someone went phishing.

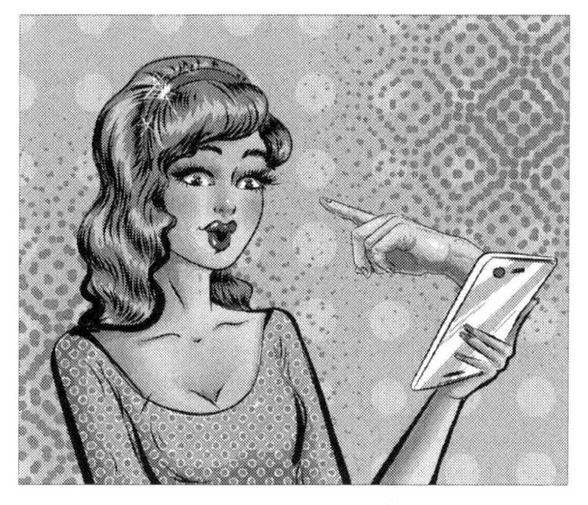

Don't believe me? Do your own experiment. And it's not just our smartphones.

Let's take home managers, or smart speakers. Apple and Google admit that Alexa and Siri spy on us. Employees listen in on conversations, but only to monitor and improve the system—or so they say. Industry claims the sampling is very small, and that they have in place strict anti-abuse regulations. (Cuthbertson, 2019)

The marriage of 5G and IoT (the Internet of Things) is one of the most insidious invasions of privacy ever promoted, and it is being implemented "under the radar."

They Locate

Even when the GPS is turned off, your location can still be established using cell tower triangulation. Although this is not exactly "pin-pointing" it can get pretty close. This could be used for good or bad, depending on who wants to know your whereabouts. (Tran, 2015)

They Log Personal Data

Your smartphone and other smart devices collect, analyze, and record thousands of interactions every day. It is no secret that this information is available to third-party advertisers. But it's for "your benefit." It's like having a "personal shopper" hunt out the best deals for you.

Google says they don't "sell" your personal information. They just place advertisements in your purview, based on your trends and search history. (Hildenbrand, 2018)

And Apple boasts on a Las Vegas over-sized billboard ahead of the Consumer Electronics Show, "What happens on your iPhone stays on your iPhone." (Miller, 2019)

However, a technology columnist begs to differ on the claims of privacy. He discovered that he was being "tracked" by third parties, and that personal information had been shared, contrary to Apple's published privacy policy. (Fowler, May 28, 2019)

What About Hackers?

In the CNET article, "Smart Homes Might be Getting too Smart. Start Worrying," the author makes the stunning point that the danger is not just that hackers could know when you are on vacation and hack your smart lock and break into your home. That's bad enough. But also there is the broader danger that hackers could commandeer hundreds of thousands of smart-phones and smart devices to request access to a bank, social media platform, or government agency, thus forcing a DDoS (Distributed Denial of Service) attack. (Priest, 2019)

This actually happened in the 2016 Mirai botnet attack that crashed the Web. (Fruhlinger, 2018)

How smart is the smart grid? In the gripping documentary film, *Take Back Your Power*, film maker Josh del Sol raises questions about privacy as well as health. The film focuses on electric utility smart meters as well as other modern appliances, and the built-in "spy" devices that are inherent in most modern appliances. And we don't even know the potential effect on our privacy.

Smart devices can be programmed to share our private information with advertisers over back-channels of which we are not aware. They ensure that Internet-enabled devices are programmed to be quite adept to share information. We can only hope that advertisements from those obtaining our personal preferences and habits is the worst-case scenario posed by this data collection. The potential for power abuse is incalculable.

The marriage of 5G and IoT (the Internet of Things) is one of the most insidious invasions of privacy ever promoted, and it is being implemented "under the radar." The telecommunications industry estimates there will be about 800,000 small cells on lamp posts, buildings, and power poles in America by 2026. However, others say it eventually could be upwards of two million of them. (Senum, 2017)

To be fair, there are some benefits to this connectivity and tracking involving safety, identifying medical emergencies, solving crimes, finding missing persons, etc. But we should not bury our heads in the sand when it comes to the issue of personal privacy. (More on 5G in Chapter 4.)

The sensors are coming.

The sensors are coming.

They've got us covered.

Do you remember the title of this chapter: Why Should You Care?

Here is the disconcerting bottom line: There are no long-term studies on the effects of EMR/EMF on humans. There are physical, mental, and social ramifications that are uncharted. We are all "guinea pigs" in a huge, highly lucrative, disorganized experiment.

Industry claims that there is no scientific proof of harm to the health of humans. Many scientists and concerned citizens suggest that there is no scientific proof that there is NOT harm to our health. Who bears the burden of proof?

Which is your particular "hot button?":

- Health and physical well-being?
- The mental and emotional health of our children?

• The uncontrollable and extensive invasion of privacy?

Why should you care?

Because there's a lot to care about. And because you are WIRED to care!

Action for Today:

✓ CARE! Have a high level of concern and keep reading.

Need or want solutions right now?

Go to Chapters 7, 8 and 9 (more than 30 pages of solutions) and Appendix I for your Comprehensive Home Safety Audit.

Chapter 2

What Is It And Where Is It?

Electro-what?

Electromagnetic radiation is known by different names:

- Electro-smog
- Electro-pollution
- Electromagnetic Fields (EMF)
- Electromagnetic Radiation (EMR)
- Dirty Electricity
- Electromagnetic Interference (EMI)
- Radio Frequency (RF)
- WiFi Radiation
- Wireless Radiation
- Bluetooth Radiation
- Electric Radiation
- Electric Fields
- Magnetic Radiation
- Magnetic Fields
- Microwave Radiation

Throughout this book I will use EMR and EMF interchangeably to refer to all of the above.

Here's what Oxford Dictionaries says:

> e·lec·tro·mag·net·ic ra·di·a·tion
> noun
> Physics: a kind of radiation including visible light, radio waves, gamma rays, and X-rays, in which electric and magnetic fields vary simultaneously.

Purcell and Morin of Harvard University explain that in physics electromagnetic radiation refers to the waves of the electromagnetic field, propagating (radiating) through space, carrying electromagnetic radiant energy. Browne further states that electromagnetic radiation includes radio waves, microwaves, infrared light, visible light, and ultraviolet light, as well as X-ray and gamma radiation.

What's the difference between the intense radiation of an X-ray and the low levels produced by modern electronics? Does it matter?

Ionizing radiation is the type of radiation that carries enough energy to break bonds between molecules and ionize atoms. Examples of Ionizing radiation are the gamma rays emitted by radioactive materials, cosmic rays, and X-rays.

Non-ionizing radiation does not carry enough energy to break molecular bonds and ionize atoms. Examples of non-ionizing are ELF (extremely low frequencies) and RF (radio-frequencies) radiation or wireless, produced by modern electronics.

When we talk about electromagnetic radiation (EMR), we are talking about non-ionizing radiation. The argument is frequently made that these levels are very LOW, and therefore not harmful. Low—right. Not harmful—wrong.

The type of EMR/EMF we are talking about is low compared to ionizing radiation, but extremely high compared to the frequencies found in nature. And extremely dangerous for long-term exposure.

I hear the argument all the time: "You get more radiation from dental X-rays or a flight in an airplane than you do from a cell phone."

The problem is that we get a constant loading of EMR in the body and it is cumulative. It is exactly the constant low levels of non-ionizing radiation that reveal metabolic changes in the body. That means the effects are seen at the cellular level.

Don't underestimate the ELF!

To simplify, let's look at it this way:
There are two types of Electromagnetic Radiation:

1. Through the Air

Wireless, WiFi, Bluetooth, and RF Radiation

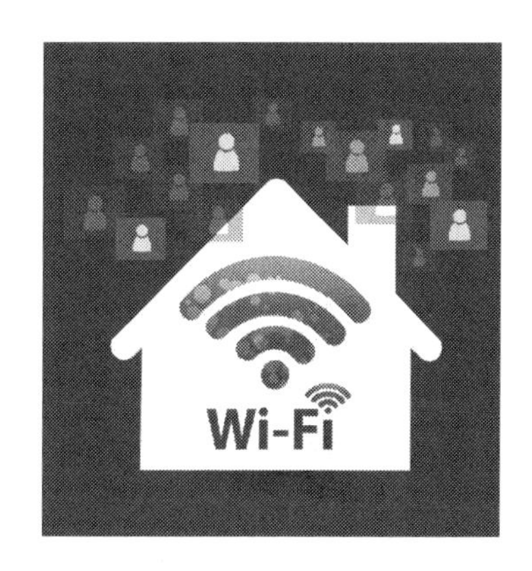

2. From the Wires

- Electric Radiation
- Magnetic Radiation
- Dirty Electricity

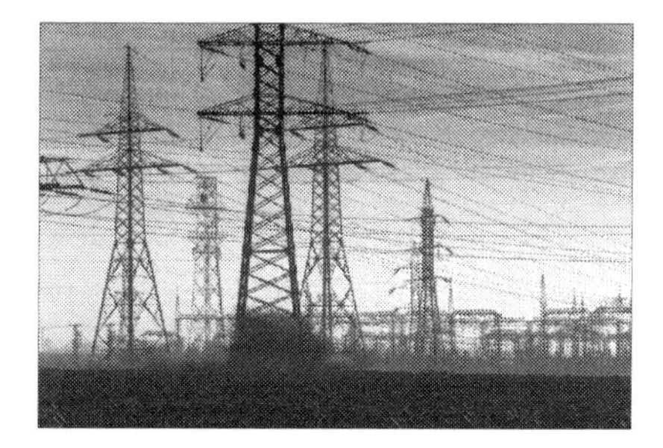

Through the Air: Wireless/WiFi/Bluetooth/RF Radiation

There is an increasing awareness of the dangers of prolonged exposure to wireless radiation. And this is the one type of radiation for which there are many simple solutions that you can implement almost immediately, for no cost. (See Section II: Chapter 8: Ten Ways to Lower Your Exposure to Harmful Radiation—Right Now!)

- Can originate inside or outside of a building.
- Most electronic devices now have a Wireless/WiFi or Bluetooth component.

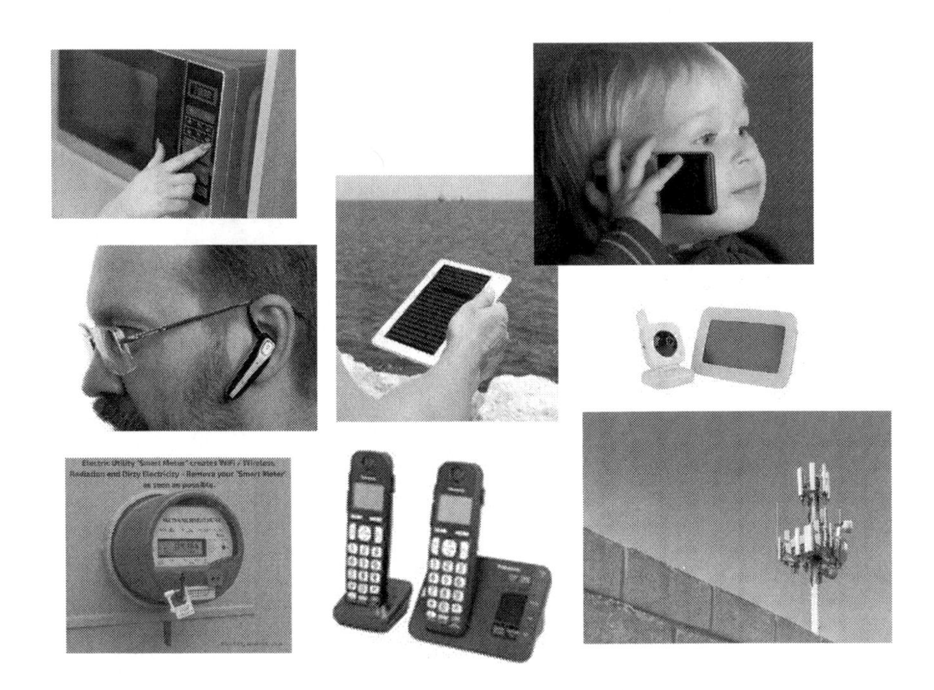

Major sources of EMR/EMF through the air include: Cell Phones – Cell Towers – Bluetooth – WiFi – Wireless – Microwave Ovens – Baby Monitors – Virtual Reality Goggles – Smart Home Devices and Systems. (See Appendix I for a comprehensive list. Solutions to wireless radiation can be found in Section II.)

I hear a lot of terms tossed around, such as WiFi/Wireless/Bluetooth, "smart," RF (radio frequency) and microwave. They are all in the category of radiation that travels through the air. They are basically the same thing. The only difference is that they use different frequencies. They all produce unsafe levels of EMR.

From Wires: Electric and Magnetic Radiation, Dirty Electricity

Electric Radiation

- Is produced by "live" electrical wires.
- It emanates from wires you can see and ones hidden behind walls—think about the wall right behind where you sleep.
- It travels 6-8 feet out from the wires.
- It exists even if the device is turned OFF.

Wait. Are you telling me that even when I turn off a lamp or appliance I'm still getting electric radiation from those wires?

Yes.

Think of a garden hose. You can turn off the water . . .

. . . but there is still water, and pressure, in the hose.

Likewise, you can turn off an electrical device, but there is still electric radiation coming from the wires.

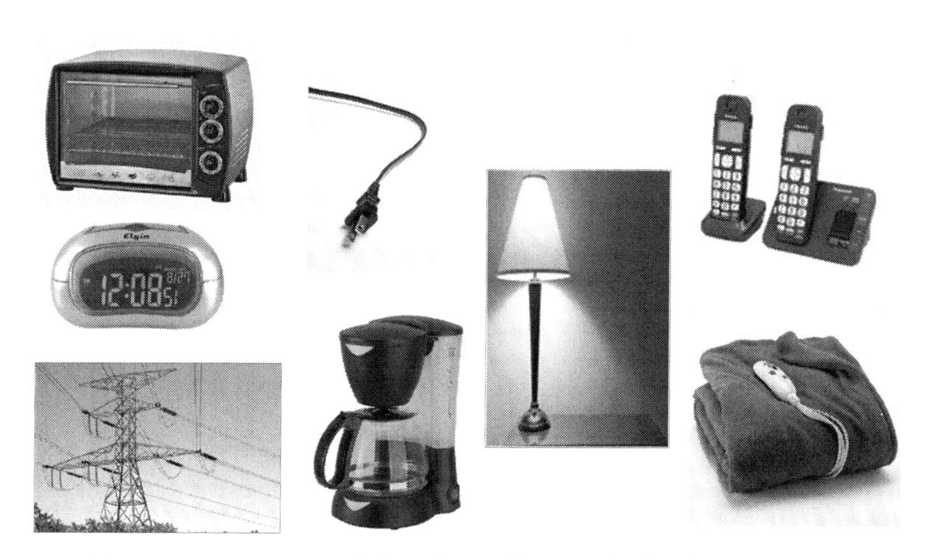

Common sources of electric radiation include: Buried Power Lines – Charging Devices – Cordless Phones – Electric Appliances – Electric Clocks – Electric Stoves – Extension Cords – House

Wiring – Laptops – Overhead Power Lines – Visible Electric Wires – on or off. (See Appendix I for a comprehensive list. Solutions for electric radiation can be found in Section II.)

Magnetic Radiation

- Is produced by the *flow* of electric current; if you have a lamp just plugged in there is electric radiation; once you turn on that lamp you have electric radiation and magnetic radiation.
- Can be found on water pipes and/or cables and TV lines entering a home.
- Can emanate 3 to 6 ft. from a wall or device in a home.
- Can travel hundreds of feet from high-voltage power lines.

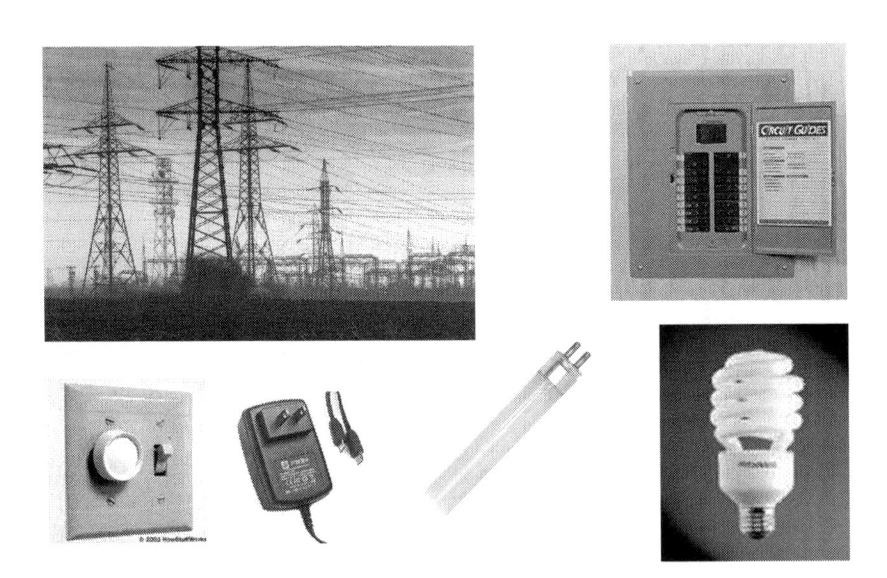

Common sources of Magnetic Radiation include:

Breaker Panels – Buried Power Lines – Chargers – Cordless Phones – Dimmer Switches – Electric Clocks – Electric Tooth Brushes – Electric Utility Meter – Freezers – Fuse Boxes – Hair Dryers – Internal Wiring errors commonly on 3-Way Switches – Energy Efficient Light Bulbs – Overhead Power lines

– Refrigerators – Stray Voltage on Water Pipes, Gas Lines, Cable TV Lines and Phone Lines. (See Appendix I for a comprehensive list. Solutions to Electric and Magnetic Radiation can be found in Section II.)

Dirty Electricity

This term is sometimes used by others generically as a synonym for the whole realm of EMR/EMF, as I have it on my website. However, dirty electricity is actually a category of its own.

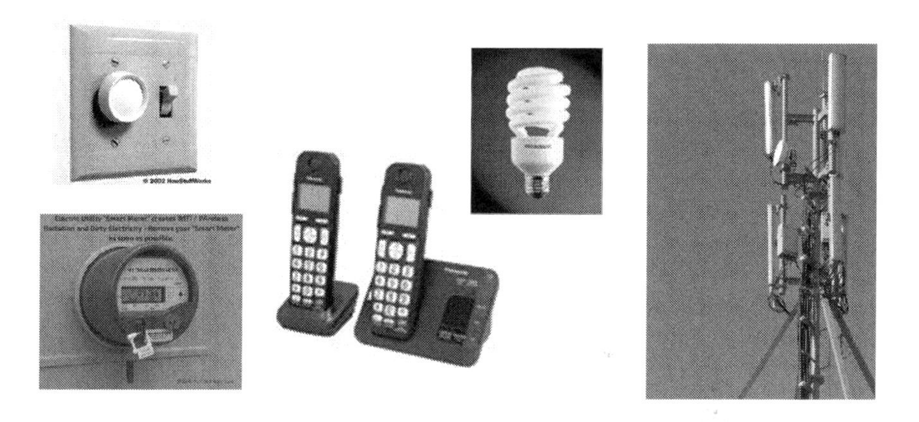

High Frequency Voltage Transients and Harmonics is the technical term for dirty electricity. It is the electrical activity that bleeds off of and rides on top of every electrical wire in your home.

The wires in your home measure at 120 volts. But most electronics run at 19 volts or less. When the electricity is “squeezed” down to 19 volts or less, it causes spikes of radiation and an “electrical aura” around every wire in your home.

Common sources of dirty electricity include: Cable Boxes – Chargers – Computers – Cordless Phones – Dimmer Switches – DVD Players – Electric Clocks – Electric Tooth Brushes – Electric Utility Meters – Electronic Devices – Freezers – Fuse Boxes – Energy Efficient Light Bulbs – Overhead Power lines – Refrigerators – Satellite Boxes – Stray Voltage on Water Pipes, Gas Lines, Cable TV Lines, Phone Lines – Televisions (See Appendix I for a comprehensive list. Solutions for Dirty Electricity can be found in Section II.)

Dirty Electricity, by its technical definition, is a controversial topic, even among electromagnetic radiation experts. In my opinion, it is a significant factor and worth taking seriously. These numbers are why. They occurred at one middle school.

24 - 49 - 12 - 13 - 10 - 9

- As many as 24 teachers and staff developed cancer.
- As many as 49 former students developed cancer.
- As many as 12 teachers, staff, and former middle school students have now died.
- 13 times the normal rate of thyroid cancer.
- 10 times the normal rate of melanoma.
- 9 times the normal rate of uterine cancer.

These numbers occurred at just ONE middle school in California. Remember when you were in your twenties? How many of your friends had cancer? And from one single middle school? Younger readers may think this is normal, because maybe it's becoming the "new normal." My wife and I can think of five people right now that we personally know who have brain tumors.

Epidemiologist Samuel Milham, MD, Master of Public Health and formerly with the State of Washington Health Department, spent his professional career studying disease and cancer clusters. He found a striking correlation between the spread of electrical services and increased cancer rates across America. (Milham, 2012)

But back to California. Dr. Milham measured some classrooms in that particular school and found the dirty electricity levels were off the charts. It was so high that it literally "pegged" the meter.

He suspected that it was coming from an electrical substation about a mile away. He offered to remediate the situation at no

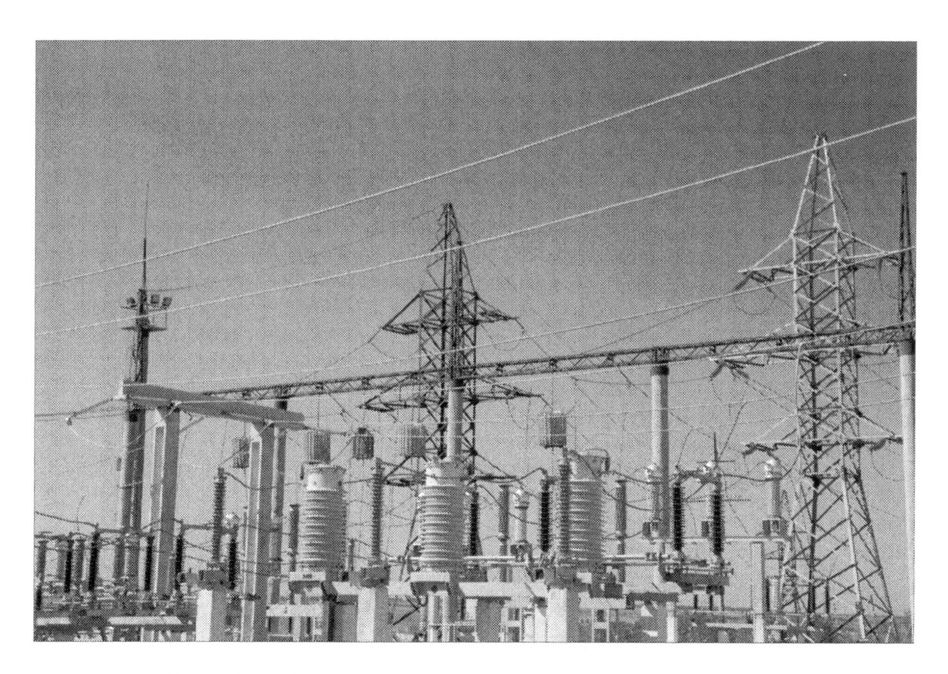

charge to the school. The next communication Dr. Milham got was from the school district's lawyers. The rest is history. A sad history indeed.

How can this happen?

Electricity runs on a circuit. Electrical wires bring it to your home, where some is used by lights and appliances. Then it returns to the power station on an accompanying wire to complete the circuit. However, it can also return through the ground. This portion of the electrical current is known as stray voltage, or stray current.

According to electrical engineer Lawrence J. Gust, BBEC, EMRS, approximately 65 percent of the current supplied by the utility returns to the generating station via the earth. "This situation is true everywhere in the U.S.," he says. (Gust, 1996)

So what's the problem? Gust further explains that electrical current in the soil produces a magnetic field and, as pointed out in Chapter 1, that electromagnetic field can cause health problems in humans and animals. Additionally, underground pipes, cables, and water sources can become conduits for that stray voltage and carry it—and its electromagnetic field—into buildings, including your home.

You might assume that stray voltage is deep underground, posing no danger to you. Not so. It runs very close to the surface of the ground, so much so that dairy farmers in the Midwest noticed that milk production in cows dramatically decreased due to cows getting shocked from ground currents. Many lawsuits have been and still are being won by dairy farmers over this issue. Muh-ooooooo! (Associated Press, 2017)

Electricity can literally travel on the surface of the ground. So, it does happen that concentrated levels of electricity can converge onto pipes and cables and enter a building, spreading electro-pollution throughout the building at excessive levels.

The change from AC (alternating current) to DC (direct current) or DC to AC also creates dirty electricity. Although AC remains the ruling standard transmission, most devices that consume electricity—cars, planes, light-rail systems, computers, consumer electronics, and pretty much anything with a battery—actually run on DC. Most electronics in your home run on 19 volts or less DC. When 120 volts AC is switched to 19 volts or less DC, spikes of radiation are generated thousands of time a second, and they "piggyback" on your electrical wiring, resulting in dirty electricity.

A similar thing happens in reverse when solar panels generate a low-voltage DC power and inverters convert this to 120 volts AC. This also results in dirty electricity. Some solar providers say their inverters are clean, but you must measure to see how much dirty electricity is being produced. Another problem with solar generation is that most systems require an additional Electric Utility Smart Meter, which generates both Dirty Electricity from the wires and wireless radiation through the air.

Another surprising source of dirty electricity is the creation of the energy-efficient light bulb. Fluorescent lights, to save energy, turn on and off 5,000 to 20,000 times per second. And modern CFLs (compact fluorescent lights—curlicue bulbs), as well as LEDs, are said to turn on and off thousands of times per second. This is indiscernible to the human eye. But the dirty electricity is measurable, and it is often off the charts. Dirty electricity is a known health hazard. So is the mercury contained in the curlicue bulbs.

So much for saving the environment.

Actions for Today:

- ✓ Realize this problem is real and all around us in many different forms.
- ✓ Begin looking for and being aware of the two types of EMR, through the AIR and from WIRES.
- ✓ Tell three friends and family about the dangers of EMR/EMF through the AIR and from WIRES.
- ✓ Keep reading and stay tuned for solutions in Section II.

Need or want solutions right now?

Go to Chapters 7, 8 and 9 (more than 30 pages of solutions) and Appendix I for your Comprehensive Home Safety Audit.

Chapter 3

*Ovem Lupo Commitere**

Is the Fine Print Really Fine?

When you purchased your last cell phone, did you read the six-point font, folded brochure that came with it? Probably not. We rarely do. We just trust that it is safe to use. So, to whom are you entrusting your health and well-being?

I took the time to read the safety instructions for both Samsung Android and Apple smartphones. You can find this information in the Samsung User Manual and the iPhone User Guide—Safety, Handling, and Support.

It was a thoroughly disappointing experience. The good and extensive research from the BioInitiative report and other sources was routinely discredited and replaced with industry-friendly citations. Point by point, it white-washed the dangers associated with wireless devices.

But, there were a few token admissions.

Did you know that the instructions from the manufacturer actually suggests, in an even smaller font size:

- ✓ Don't put the mobile device directly up to your ear.
- ✓ Don't carry the mobile device in a breast pocket.
- ✓ Use common sense to avoid situations where your skin is in contact with a device or its power adapter when it's operating or plugged into a power source for long periods of time. For example, don't sleep with or place a

---

* To entrust a wolf to guard sheep

device or power adapter under a blanket, pillow, or next to your body when it's plugged into a power source.

See the Dr. Gupta interview conducted by CNN's Anderson Cooper: "Cell Phone Radiation Safety Tips": YouTube.com/watch?v=v7wCeuSqm34.

But the industry guidelines are based on some disturbing and short-sighted assumptions.

Do You Know the Difference Between SAR and SAM?

Industry claims the SAR (specific absorption rate) proves its safety. Did you know that the research was based on SAM? SAM is an acronym for Standard Anthropomorphic Man, also called Anthropometric. And sometimes referred to as Specific Anthropomorphic Mannequin. He's a BFD! A Big Fake Dummy.

SAM was a 6'2", 220-pound dummy representing the top ten percent of U.S. military recruits in 1989. He was given an 11-pound hollow head, about the size of a bowling ball, filled with various liquids. His cell phone usage was about SIX minutes a day. Whom do you know that fits those criteria? (Gandhi et al., 2011; Davis, 2013; DeBaun & DeBaun, 2017)

How does this SAR rate translate to a real human body? And what about a pregnant woman or a small child?

There's a BIG problem with SAM.

He represents only the largest three percent of cell phone users since his head size is based upon a 6'2" man weighing 220 pounds. So, if a cell phone emits radiation into SAM's head at the maximum level allowed by the FCC, that same phone could expose 97 percent of us to greater radiation than the federal FCC emission standards allow. (Consumers For Safe Phones, 2011; Natural Society, retrieved 2017)

This is a VERY serious issue for the smallest and most vulnerable of cell phone users—children. Additionally, industry touts that cell phones expose us to very low levels of radiation.

If you recall some of the research cited in Chapter 1, it was exactly *low levels* of radiation that caused DNA strands to break, compromised the blood-brain barrier, and brought observable challenges to the immune system at the cellular level.

Moreover, industry guidelines recommend the use of an ear piece. Think about that. Where do most people carry their phones while using an ear piece? On their belt? In their pocket? Internal organs are still getting all the exposure to radiation that the head would have gotten. So, save the brain and fry your kidneys? (Radiant Insights, 2016)

And would that ear piece be wired or wireless? What are the benefits and risks? No mention.

Who is watching this soon-to-be trillion-dollar industry in

The key insight is that industry doesn't have to win the scientific argument about safety; it only has to keep the argument going.

---

the USA? Internationally, it's already over $2 trillion.

The FCC. The Federal Communications Commission. If you go to its website and click on, "What We Do," you will find that the FCC serves industry. It has little to do with health and safety. The FCC was originally created to bring fairness to business. If New York had a wireless infrastructure in place, but New Jersey did not, wouldn't that give New York an unfair commercial advantage? So, the FCC has served an important commercial purpose. But it is neither equipped for nor interested in seriously addressing issues of health and safety.

The FCC does from time to time have to answer questions. And whom does the FCC appoint as expert witnesses? People from the very industry that stands to gain tremendous amounts of money. (Hertsgaard & Dowie, 2018)

The key insight is that industry doesn't have to win the scientific argument about safety; it only has to keep the argument going. That amounts to a win for the industry, because the apparent lack of certainty helps to reassure customers and fend off government regulations.

Sadly, there are some real-life testimonies of industry "expert witnesses" who bamboozle courtrooms with "scientific mumbo-jumbo" and discredit and humiliate those who present the honest scientific research. If you don't believe me, read for yourself:

- *Going Somewhere—Truth About a Life in Science* by Andrew Marino, PhD, JD, or
- *Corporate Ties That Bind—An Examination of Corporate Manipulation and Vested Interest in Public Health*, edited by Martin J. Walker, or
- *Cross Currents: The Perils of Electropollution, the Promise of Electromedicine* by Robert O. Becker, or
- Paul Brodeur's *Currents of Death – Power Lines, Computer Terminals, and the Attempt to Cover up Their Threats to Your Health.* (See Appendix II.)

Who exerts the influence?

In politics, the "revolving door" is a movement of personnel between roles as legislators and regulators and the industries affected by the legislation. According to Oxford Dictionaries, the term is used to refer to someone who moves from an influential government position to a position in a private company, or vice versa. There is a "revolving door" between politicians and lobbyists that is traceable.

The Center for Responsive Politics' Revolving Door project intends to identify those people whose career trajectory has taken them from Capitol Hill, the White House, and Cabinet office suites to "K Street," a street in Washington, DC, where many lobbyists traditionally have offices. The Center's Revolving Door database is the most comprehensive source to date to help the public learn who's who in the Washington influence industry, and to uncover how these lobbyists' government connections buy their clients privileged access to those in power. (Visit opensecrets.org.)

We need to research the research and follow the dollars. The average person doesn't have the time to do that. That's why I wrote this book.

A Walk Down Memory Lane—Asbestos, BPA, Formaldehyde, Lead, Pesticides, Tobacco

The best predictor of the future is the past. Let's look at the track record of industries and the government agencies that were supposed to keep us safe.

Remember the list in Chapter 1 of things we once thought were safe?

Asbestos:

Take a deep breath.

- 1918: The U.S. Government recognizes the risk of asbestos to human health.
- 1934: The link between cancer and workplace asbestos exposure is discovered.
- 1930s–1950s: Documents reveal that asbestos manufacturers were aware of the health risks related to exposure to asbestos but they chose to conceal this information from their employees. (MesotheliomaHelp, retrieved 2018; Barbalace, 2004)
- 1960s: There are more than 200 publications describing the health hazards of asbestos. Industry and government agencies largely ignore the medical literature.

> Today: Despite the severity of asbestos-related diseases, the material has extremely widespread use in many areas. The continuing long-term use of asbestos after harmful health effects were known or suspected, and the slow emergence of symptoms decades after that exposure had ended, makes asbestos litigation the longest, most expensive mass tort in U.S. history. (Tweedale, 2017)

The government knows asBESTos."

BPA plastics ("bisphenol A")

BPA is an industrial chemical that has been used to make certain plastics.

How Many Baby Bottles Does It Take?

- 1930s: The first evidence of BPA toxicity emerges. Scientists discover that BPA is an artificial estrogen.
- 1988: It is discovered that the EPA's safety standard for BPA is up to 25 times higher than harmful levels.
- 1997: Government tests reveal BPA contamination in infant formula.
- 1999: BPA is found to leach from baby bottles. But the FDA publicly asserts the safety thereof, claiming that low levels of BPA are not harmful.
- 2003-2006: The risk assessment for BPA as a possible reproductive and developmental toxin is evaluated. Problem is, industry consultants are tied to the research and they hand pick the government advisory panel.
- 2007: Industry influence on BPA science is revealed and challenged, and Congress investigates.
- 2008: The government finally finds that BPA poses serious health risks to humans. Walmart and other retailers pull BPA products from shelves.
- 2011: An international movement on BPA in baby bottles arises.

(Houlihan et al., 2008; Vogel, 2009; Caliendo, 2012; FDA, 2014; Bauer, retrieved 2018)

After about 90 years I think we can agree to be BPA-free.

Formaldehyde:

What's that smell?

When you think of formaldehyde, it may conjure up memories of high school biology class, and those dreaded large jars with pink things in them. But it is more than just a lab compound. It is with us in household and personal-care products, plywood, adhesives, and even some fabrics. In fact, the next time you buy new furniture or install new cabinets, be sure to open all the windows. That out-gassing smell is likely to be formaldehyde.

- 1987: The U.S. Environmental Protection Agency (EPA) classified formaldehyde as a probable human carcinogen under conditions of unusually high or prolonged exposure.

  Fact sheets from U.S. government agencies—Occupational Safety and Health Administration, Environmental Protection Agency, Centers for Disease Control and Prevention—and also a "Formaldehyde and Cancer Risk" fact sheet from the National Cancer Institute, all detail the health risks associated with formaldehyde.

  Formaldehyde has been classified as a known human carcinogen by the International Agency on Research on Cancer and by the U.S. National Toxicology Program.

  Yet, the chemical industry responds to these reports by successfully lobbying for a follow-up study. Safety regulations are delayed by downplaying the risks and questioning the science, resulting in endless reviews, endless reviews, endless reviews.
- 2017: Apparently, lobbying is the name of the game. According to the Open Secrets 2017 Summary, taken from the Senate Office of Public Records, the chemical industry continues to be a major money force for lobbying:
  - Total for Chemical & Related Manufacturing: $52,251,297
  - Total Number of Clients Reported: 108
  - Total Number of Lobbyists Reported: 426
  - Total Number of Revolvers: 261 (61.3%)

  State-level Lobbying—membership in American Legislative Exchange Council provides the American

Chemistry Council (ACC) with added access to lawmakers and the ability to influence the development and passage of state policies directly. (U.S. House of Representatives, 2008; Sapien, 2008; Blum, 2012; OpenSecrets.org, retrieved 2018; National Cancer Institute, retrieved 2018)

Call me formalde-phobic, but this makes my skin burn.

Lead in Paints:

- 400 BC: Hippocrates accurately described the symptoms of lead poisoning.
- 1950s: How do toddlers explore their world? With an open mouth.

  Pediatrician and child psychiatrist Herbert Needleman made the connection between lead in paint and neurological disorders when he discovered that some of the children he was treating had been chewing on paint chips and breathing fumes from badly peeling walls in enclosed areas.

  Lead is a highly toxic chemical, with lead-based paint regarded as the most identifiable hazard. If a child eats paint chips, or spends a lot of time breathing paint fumes, it could cause seizures, learning disabilities, coma, and even death.
- 1978: Decades later, lead-containing paints were finally banned and phased out.

Bypass the chips, please.

Lead in Gasoline:

- 1922: Lead was first introduced into gasoline, immediately drawing headlines concerning public health.
- 1996: It wasn't until almost 75 years later that use in all on-road vehicles was eventually completely banned.

There was, and still is, a whole lot of moneyed influence being pumped into our government.

OpenSecrets.org 2019 Summary for Lobbying:

- Total for Oil & Gas: more than $124 million.
- Total Number of Clients Reported: 190.
- Total Number of Lobbyists Reported: 699.
- Total Number of Revolvers: 490 (66.7%).

(Center for Responsive Politics, 2020)

When it came to safety issues, they ran this lap as if they had lead in their pants.

Pesticides:

"-cide" words. Have you ever noticed what suicide, genocide, fungicide, homicide, infanticide, and pesticide all have in common? The "-cide" suffix, which comes from the Latin, evokes death and destruction.

Pesticides have been around for thousands of years in the form of smoke, various plant extracts such as bitter lupin or wild cucumber, Pyrethrum daisies, and even arsenic.

We will look at several closely related chemicals: DDT, DES, and Dioxin. All are toxic in small quantities. All dissolve and accumulate in fat cells. None of them degrade in the environment—they exist indefinitely once released.

What do pests, potatoes, procreation, and paper plates have in common?

- 1939: A chemist in Switzerland developed a new compound that would profoundly change the lives of farmers around the globe. Paul Muller demonstrated that DDT killed the Colorado potato beetle, a pest that was ravaging the potato crops across America and Europe.

  DDT quickly became the new "wonder insecticide" and was credited with saving thousands of human lives in World War II by killing typhus-carrying lice and malaria-carrying mosquitoes. In fact, Paul Muller is awarded a Nobel Prize in medicine for discovering the insect-killing properties of DDT.

In the years to come, this wonder chemical turned from a savior to a scourge. DDT was eventually banned. But it took a very long time.

- 1950s: DDT is shown to disrupt sexual development in roosters. Scientists V.F. Lindeman and Howard Burlington find that young roosters treated with DDT fail to develop normal male sex characteristics, such as combs and wattles. The pesticide also stunted the growth of the animals' testes. These scientists noted a similarity between DDT and DES, a synthetic estrogen given to women for problem pregnancies.
- 1962: *Silent Spring* is published. Rachel Carson's book describes health problems observed in wildlife, such as egg shell thinning, deformities, and population declines. Carson links these adverse effects to exposure to pesticides and other synthetic chemicals.
- 1972: The newly formed EPA issues a cancellation order for the agricultural use of DDT based on its adverse environmental effects upon wildlife, as well as its potential human health risks.
- 1976: DES (synthetic estrogen) is shown to cause developmental abnormalities in male mice and reproductive problems in humans.
- 1985: The National Dioxin Survey is completed.

  But research by Greenpeace and other activist groups uncovers collusion between EPA and the paper bleaching industry to keep secret the detection of dioxin in discharges from paper mills and in finished paper products. Under threat of lawsuit, EPA releases National Dioxin Survey. The study finds dioxin is present in discharge from paper mills and in finished paper products (due to chlorine bleaching of paper). (Van Strum & Merrell, 1987)

  Leaked documents from the American Paper Institute reveal industry's strategy to "Get EPA to 'rethink' dioxin risk assessment" so as to avoid liability and "unnecessary changes" in production processes prompted by "unsound scientific data." (Weisskopf, 1987)

- 1990: The Chlorine Institute, starts a public campaign claiming that dioxin is "much less toxic to humans than originally believed," misrepresenting scientific opinion on its dangers. (*NEJM,* retrieved 2018)

  And the expected government response is? ddddddddddddd (drum roll) EPA administrator Bill Reilly tells *The New York Times*: "We are now seeing new information on dioxin that suggests a lower risk assessment for dioxin should be applied." EPA launches its second reassessment of di*oxin.* (Portier, 1993; EPA, 2003; Environmental Working Group, 2010; Lah, 2011; PBS Frontline, retrieved 2018)
- Today: Nearly 40 years after DDT was banned for use in agriculture, we continue to live with its long-lasting effects:

  Food supplies: The USDA found DDT breakdown products in 60 percent of heavy cream samples, 42 percent of kale greens, 28 percent of carrots, and lower percentages of many other foods.

  Production, use, and management: DDT is currently being produced in three countries: India, China, and North Korea. By far the largest amounts are produced in India for the purpose of disease control. (Carlson, 1962; Brooks & Roberts, 2003; Banaszkiewicz, 2010; Hardell, 2017)

How long **DiD** it **T**ake?

Tobacco and smoking:

We're going to get off Memory Lane now and take a turn down Smoke Alley.

Tobacco smoking has been around for a long time, initially smoked in pipes and as cigars, and later as hand-rolled cigarettes. But in 1883, James Bonsack invented a machine that could roll cigarettes and produce thousands per day. Bonsack began a business called the American Tobacco Company, which was the first company to produce cigarettes on a large scale. This invention changed the stage forever.

For a fascinating, highly detailed time line of tobacco-related events, go to Tobacco News and Information, Tobacco Timeline: archive.tobacco.org/History/Tobacco_History.html. See Appendix III for links to additional tobacco timelines.

The history of tobacco will light you up and get you on a long, slow burn. Here are just a few of the low points in the tobacco industry saga taken from the above sources:

- 1929: Fritz Lickint of Dresden publishes the first formal statistical evidence of a lung cancer-tobacco link, based on cases showing that lung cancer sufferers were likely to be smokers.
- 1930s: Fritz Lickint, in collaboration with the Reich Committee for the Struggle against Addictive Drugs and the German Antitobacco League, publishes Tobacco and the Organism. Dr. Robert Proctor, Professor of the History of Sciences, Stanford University, calls the 1,100-page volume "arguably the most comprehensive scholarly indictment of tobacco ever published." It blamed smoking for cancers all along the "smoke alley"—lips, tongue, mouth, jaw, esophagus, windpipe, and lungs, and even included a warning about what we call today, "second-hand smoke."

  Franz Muller presents the world's first controlled epidemiological study of the tobacco-lung cancer relationship, "Tobacco Misuse and Lung Carcinoma." The research finds that "the extraordinary rise in tobacco use [is] the single most important cause of the rising incidence of lung cancer." (Proctor, 1999)

- 1940s: Much of the research is done in Germany. What's happening in the U.S.? JAMA (Journal of the American Medical Association) publishes articles linking smoking with a higher risk of coronary disease and lung cancer, while the AMA itself participates in a Camel exhibit at an R.J. Reynolds convention.

  What's the difference between, AMA and JAMA? Just the "J."

  R. J. Reynolds (RJR) launches "More Doctors Smoke Camels" ad campaign.
- 1950s: Tobacco companies continue to assert that smoking is completely harmless. But just in case, the "Micronite" filter is offered as "the greatest health protection in cigarette history." Its secret? Asbestos.

  That's right. Doctors in their white coats and stethoscopes are shown on TV, pleasantly puffing a cigarette.

  Dr. Ernst L. Wynder's landmark report finds that painting cigarette tar on the backs of mice creates tumors. This was the first successful induction of cancer in a lab animal with a tobacco product, and the first definitive biological link between smoking and cancer.

  In December 1953, the president of the American Tobacco Company and the CEOs of the biggest tobacco companies in America gathered to develop a strategic response to the scientific research that revealed the link between cigarette smoking and lung cancer and the subsequent "health scare." They formed the Tobacco Industry Research Committee (TIRC) and worked with a high-powered public relations firm to distribute its propaganda.

The TIRC immediately ran a full-page promotion in more than 400 newspapers reaching an estimated 43 million Americans. That piece was titled "A Frank Statement To Cigarette Smokers" (See the adjacent sidebar.)

- 1960s: The American Medical Association (AMA) accepts a $10 million grant for tobacco research from six cigarette companies and delays any official word on smoking and health for another 10 years. Cha-ching!

  The AMA ends with this statement: "We are pledging aid and assistance to the research effort into all phases of tobacco use and health." From *The Facts About Smoking* (Consumer Reports Books,1992) After lulling the public into a false sense of security concerning smoking and health, the Tobacco Industry Research Committee continues to speak for tobacco industry interests. In spite of the initial public statements and posturing, there was a coordinated, industry-wide strategy designed to actively mislead and confuse the public about the true dangers associated with smoking cigarettes.

  There is no question that the tobacco industry knew what the scientific research revealed about tobacco. But they kept the fake controversy alive with a carefully selected 18-page booklet titled, "A Scientific Perspective on the Cigarette Controversy," which was mailed to more than 200,000 people, including doctors, members of Congress, and the news media. (White, 1988; Cummings et al., 2002)

PAUSE:

Are you wondering where our government was in all of this? Me, too.

continued on page 58

A Frank Statement to Cigarette Smokers

Introductory note: In December 1953, Paul M. Hahn, president of the American Tobacco Co., and the CEOs of the biggest tobacco companies in America, met to develop a response to scientific research that revealed the link between cigarette smoking and lung cancer.

Under the guise of their newly formed "research" committee, these industry leaders ran a full-page promotion, titled "A Frank Statement to Cigarette Smokers," in hundreds of newspapers nationwide. Below are the key points of the advertisement. See if you recognize any familiar phrases. Feel free to plug in your words of choice within the brackets.

- Recent reports on experiments with mice have given wide publicity to the theory that [*cigarette smoking*] is in some way linked with [*lung*] cancer in human beings.
- These experiments are not regarded as conclusive in the field of cancer research.
- There is no agreement among the authorities regarding the cause of [*lung*] cancer.
- No proof that [*cigarette smoking*] is one of the causes.
- We believe our products are not injurious to health.
- For more than [*300*] years [*tobacco*] has given solace, relaxation, and enjoyment to mankind. At one time or another during those years, critics have held it responsible for practically every disease of the human body. One by one these charges have been abandoned for lack of evidence.

The statement was signed by the major companies producing tobacco products and the companies' presidents.

To read the entire statement, go to:
sourcewatch.org/index.php/The_Frank_Statement

Congressman John Blatnik headed a commission on smoking and the report was delivered to Congress. "The cigarette manufacturers have deceived the American public through their advertising of filter-tip cigarettes. . . . The Federal Trade Commission has failed in its statutory duty to 'prevent deceptive acts or practice' in filter-cigarette advertising."

Very shortly afterward, Blatnik's commission went up in smoke. (Cummings & Proctor, 2014)

- 1960: FDA expresses its interpretation that tobacco does not fit the "hazardous" criteria stated in the Federal Hazardous Substances Labeling Act (FHSA) of 1960.

  Sadly, tobacco companies continue to win law suits, even though they know very early on that nicotine is a drug and that smoking was linked to cancer and other diseases.

  Cigarettes are the most heavily advertised product in America.
- 1965: The Federal Cigarette Labeling and Advertising Act of 1965 (Public Law 89–92) required that the warning "Caution: Cigarette Smoking May Be Hazardous to Your Health" be placed in small print on one of the side panels of each cigarette package. The act ***prohibited*** additional labeling requirements at the federal, state, or local levels.
- 1970s: Tobacco companies purchase and control their own research companies.

  President Nixon signs a measure banning cigarette advertising on radio and television.

  Cigarette ads are taken off TV and radio as the Cigarette Smoking Act of 1969 takes effect. The last commercial on U.S. TV is a Virginia Slims ad, aired on Johnny Carson's Tonight Show, just before the Jan. 1, 1971, ban.

  The Tobacco Institute memo describes the industry's strategy for defending itself in litigation, politics, and public opinion as "brilliantly conceived and executed over the years" in order to "cast doubt about the health charge" by using "variations on the theme that 'the case is not proved.'" The memo urges more intensive lobbying.

Nixon Administration Surgeon General Dr. Jesse Steinfeld is fired after angering tobacco executives by urging restrictions on second-hand smoke.

The Tobacco Institute concludes that the nonsmokers' rights movement is "the most dangerous development yet to the viability of the tobacco industry . . ."

- 1980s: Surgeon General (C. Everett Koop) calls nicotine "a powerfully addicting drug." In his office's 618-page summary of more than 2,000 studies of nicotine and its effects on the body, Koop declares, "It is now clear that . . . cigarettes and other forms of tobacco are addicting and that actions of nicotine provide the pharmacologic basic of tobacco addiction."

  Courts across the country find evidence of a conspiracy by tobacco companies to deceive the public.
- 1990s: The winds shift and smoking begins to waft out.

  Individuals and groups going to court against tobacco companies start to win. Finally.

  Smoking bans are instituted in restaurants, post offices, libraries, airplanes, cruise ships, and military buildings.

  The Environmental Protection Agency (EPA) declares cigarette smoke a Class-A carcinogen.

  Tobacco companies shift to the concern about second-hand smoke and their cronies try to dismiss it as being inconsequential. *Consumers' Research Magazine* (July 1991) publishes the article "Passive Smoking: How Great a Hazard?" by Gary L. Huber, Robert E. Brockie, and Vijay K Mahajan. The authors—all three of them medical doctors who also published a book of the same title—claim that "ETS [environmental tobacco smoke] is so highly diluted that it is not even appropriate to call it smoke." (Borio, 2001)

Scientists from Canada report finding evidence of cigarette smoke in fetal hair, the first biochemical proof that the offspring of non-smoking mothers can be affected by passive cigarette smoke. (Eliopoulos et al., 1994)

A *New York Times* front-page article reveals "secret" tobacco papers. (*Mother Jones*, May/June 1996; Bates & Rowell, 1998)

FDA declares nicotine a drug. (White, 1988; Kennedy & Berob, 1999; Proctor, 2012; Ruff, 2017)

For a smooth taste of nicotine propaganda, check out the 1972 film produced by the tobacco industry. Notice how they create doubt, disparage good research, and divert attention, claiming that stress and genetics rather than smoking causes illness: "Smoking and Health: The Need to Know" [archive.org/details/tobacco_hjy99d00].

The EMR issue, unlike previous hazards, has a worldwide foothold with enormous monetary and social power, accompanied by high customer approval.

Smoke and mirrors: The obscuring or embellishing of the truth of a situation with misleading or irrelevant information.

So, to whom shall we entrust our health? We are prone to want to hear good news about our bad habits. And when industry-friendly scientists, along with government agencies, are not alarmed into action, it's easy to buy into that false sense of security.

The government's track record looks hazy at best.

And Now We Add EMR

Electromagnetic radiation:

If you have endured the painful history of things that were said to be "safe" but were really dangerous, I think you can reasonably conclude that neither industry nor government agencies are on the front line, watching out for our health. Would you expect different results for the Telecommunications Industry and governmental agencies such as the FCC?

Only it's worse. The EMR issue, unlike previous hazards, has a worldwide foothold with enormous monetary and social power, accompanied by high customer approval. In other words, we love and depend upon our technology more than we've ever loved or depended upon smoking, BPA, asbestos, pesticides, leaded paint and gasoline, etc. And it's a universal dependence. Business and social connections piggyback on technology all around the world. We love our technology. Why would we want to listen to naysayers about something that rings our chimes so perfectly?

How did it all start?

- 1746: The genie is let out of the bottle by Pieter van Musschenbroek, professor of physics at the University of Leyden, The Netherlands. He spins the glass bottle and rubs it, drawing out static electricity that sparks fascination and obsession all over Europe.

  This results in everything from serious scientific experimentation to party tricks and "electric kisses." Medical experimentation abounds and is directed at deafness, heart rate, blood flow, and mental illness, to name only a few. (Firstenberg, 2017)
- 1747: Benjamin Franklin (along with others) begins conducting a series of electrical experiments that make him a household name around the world. He discovers what we today call a positive or negative charge.

- 1752: The famous "Kite Experiment" by Benjamin Franklin and colleagues.
- 1780: Luigi Galvini discovers he can make the leg of a frog twitch when he applies electricity to it.
- 1819: The Danish physicist Hans Christian Oersted notes that a compass needle moves in the presence of an electric field, thus establishing the fundamental relationship between electricity and magnetism. We call the entire field electromagnetics.
- 1831: Michael Faraday demonstrates electromagnetic induction and builds the first direct-current generator. (Mathias, 2004)
- 1864: James Clerk Maxwell proves the existence of electromagnetic waves.
- 1876: Thomas Edison creates the first industrial research laboratory. His inventions include: electric incandescent light bulb, power utilities, batteries, sound recording, and motion pictures. Edison's inventions contribute to mass communication.
- 1880s: Edison develops a system of electric power generation and distribution to homes, businesses, and factories—a crucial development in the modern industrialized world.
- 1887: Heinrich Hertz invents the oscillator (an alternating-current generator) and creates radio waves.
- Late 1880s: Thomas Edison and Nikola Tesla become embroiled in a battle now known as the War of the Currents. Experiments and research continue and the battle over AC (alternating current) and DC (direct current) escalate. Interestingly, Edison strongly opposes the use of AC.
- The electrification of Europe and the United States begins and spreads rapidly.
- 1889: Power lines spread all across Europe and the U.S.
- 1892: Thomas Edison's institutional opposition to

alternating current comes to an end when he merges his company with what had become his biggest competitor, the Thomson-Houston Company. The merger puts the managers of Thomson-Houston in control of the new company, called General Electric.

There are several technical factors that drove the adoption of alternating-current over direct-current.

1. The direct-current system generated and distributed electrical power at the same voltage as used by the customer's lamps and motors. This required the use of large, costly distribution wires.

2. With the development of the transformer, alternating-current power could be sent long distances over relatively small wires at a high voltage, then reduced in voltage to that used by a customer. Alternating-current generating stations could be larger and more efficient, and the distribution wires were less costly. The lower cost of AC power distribution prevailed.

- 1899: Guglielmo Marconi sends a radio telegraph transmission across the English Channel, and in 1901 a transmission across the Atlantic.

PAUSE:

Are there any reported health concerns swirling around this new-found genie? Yes. Many early pioneers of electricity reported alarming health issues, including paralysis, tremors, headaches, stroke, vertigo, eye-sight problems, and many more. Granted, some were involved in heavy doses under bizarre circumstances. But still. (Firstenberg, 2017)

ONWARD:

- 1920s: Radio is the new rage. Public radio broadcasts spring up. Police cars use radio dispatch communication.
- 1930s: TV is introduced in Europe and the U.S.

The FCC (Federal Communications Commission) begins and takes over wire communication regulation from the Interstate Commerce Commission.

Radar is invented.

- 1940s: The first commercial mobile radiotelephone service is introduced in St. Louis. Engineers at Bell Labs develop the concept of cellular technology.

  The transistor is invented by Nobel Prize winning scientists John Bardeen, Walter Brattain, and William Shockley. The transistor serves as the foundation for the development of modern electronics and the use of computers and communications.
- 1950s: The first microwave telecommunication system is installed to support 2,400 telephone circuits.

  Radar is further developed by the military.
- 1960s: The first communication satellite, Telstar, is launched into orbit.

  The International Telecommunications Satellite Consortium (INTELSAT) is established.

  The Advanced Research Projects Agency (ARPA) develops the precursor of the modern Internet.

  The FCC opens Docket 18262 to set aside sufficient spectrum to meet the demand for land mobile communications. Congestion on the frequencies then available had approached unacceptable levels, with a waiting period of several years to get a mobile phone.
- 1970s: FCC authorizes cellular systems launch in Chicago and the Washington, DC/Baltimore region.

  RESEARCH: EMR is shown to compromise the blood-brain barrier. (Oscar and Hawkins, 1977; Frey, 1979)

  RESEARCH: Epidemiologist Nancy Wertheimer looks for possible causes for a number of childhood leukemia cases in the Denver, Colorado, metropolitan area (1979). Her research, performed with physicist Ed

Leeper, finds that children with leukemia are more than twice as likely to have lived in homes near high-voltage power lines, where the electromagnetic fields are stronger. This prompted additional research in the following decades.

RESEARCH: Russians do extensive research and testing of EMFs.

- 1980s: Motorola introduces the first truly "mobile" radiotelephone, called the "brick."

IBM PC: Low-cost assemblage of electronic parts bring computers to every small office and home.

The Cellular Telecommunications Industry Association is founded.

The FCC releases the ISM (Industrial, Scientific and Medical) band for unlicensed use, paving the way for wireless local-area networking, commonly known as LAN.

One millionth cellular subscriber is added in October 1987.

FCC's Auxiliary Cellular Services Order adopts technical flexibility rules for cellular radio without mandating specific standards, which promotes the introduction of advanced cellular technologies by the industry.

The Motorola MicroTAC is introduced, the smallest and lightest phone available at the time, weighing 12.3 ounces.

RESEARCH: Lots of interest in EMF by scientists—David Savitz, Andrew Marino, Robert Becker, to name only a few. *The New Yorker* staff writer Paul Brodeur's book, *Currents of Death: Power Lines, Computer Terminals and the Attempt to Cover Up Their Threat to Your Health* hits newsstands.

Dr. Robert Becker publishes the book, *The Body Electric: Electromagnetism and the Foundation of Life.*

(Marino, AIBS, 1985; Marino & Morris, 1985; Marino, 1986; Marino, 1987; Savitz & Calle, 1987; Marino, 1988; Savitz et al., 1988; Savitz et al., 1989; Marino, 1993; Eby, 2006)

PAUSE:

This industry is about to exPLODE. And so does the research regarding public health concerns. I'm not even going to attempt to list all of the research, as other books, along with the *BioInitiative 2012* report, do that. (See Appendices II and III.)

ONWARD:

- 1990: Cellular subscribership surpasses 5 million.
- 1991: One of the earliest "browsers" was introduced by Tim Berners-Lee and HyperText Markup Language (HTML), becomes the common language of the World Wide Web.

  RESEARCH: The biological effects of Extremely Low Frequencies (ELF) continue to be studied.
- 1992: The number of cellular users passes the 10 million milestone.

  One-millionth host connected to the Internet, with the size approximately doubling every year.

  Email takes off.
- 1993: Congress adopts the Omnibus Budget Reconciliation Act of 1993, which establishes wireless regulation and authorizes the FCC to auction spectrum for the first time.

  The first smartphone—IBM's Simon—is released to the public and offers consumers a calendar, address book, calculator, email, faxing services, and games.
- 1994: FCC begins licensing Personal Communication Services (PCS) spectrum (1.7 to 2.3 GHz). The license auction raises $7.7 billion for the U.S. Treasury.

  Cha-ching!

RESEARCH: More studies confirm that EMR affects brain function. (Bell et al., 1994)

- 1995: Windows 95.
- 1996: The Telecommunications Act of 1996 becomes law, in part designed to open other communications markets to competition. ***It states that the placement of a cell phone tower can never be denied based on health or environmental concerns.*** It also restricts local governments or individuals from impeding the spread of telecommunications infrastructure.

  RESEARCH: Electromagnetic fields, cancer, and the theory of neuroendocrine-related promotion. (Marino, 1993)

  RESEARCH: Single- and double-strand DNA breaks in rat brain cells after acute exposure to radio-frequency electromagnetic radiation. (Lai, 1996)
- 1997: The wireless industry unveils its "Safety—Your Most Important Call" to help educate drivers about the dangers of distracted driving.

  Balanced Budget Act of 1997 calls for auctioning additional commercial spectrum.
- 1998: Google becomes super popular; usage skyrockets.
- 1999: WiFi brand is adopted for technology based upon Institute of Electrical and Electronics Engineers (IEEE) specifications for wireless local-area networking.

  With the Wireless Communications and Public Safety Act of 1999, Congress designates 911 as the universal emergency number of wire line and wireless service and promotes the use of technologies that help public safety service providers locate wireless 911 callers.

  Blackberry enters the scene. Used by the government, and others.

  RESEARCH: Dr. George Carlo, a medical scientist and epidemiologist and chief scientist of the world's largest research effort into wireless safety from 1993 to 1999, heads Wireless Technologies Research, LLC, a $28.5 million research program funded by the cellular phone industry that investigated the possible health effects of cellular phones. Studies initially found that there were no significant health threats posed by such devices. But research continued, and by 1999, Dr. Carlo had changed his mind. He was convinced by the scientific evidence that health threats (including the chromosome damage, leakage of the blood-brain barrier, and cancers of the auditory nerve) were in fact linked to EMR.

- 2000: The Cellular Telecommunications Industry Association merges with the Wireless Data Forum to become the Cellular Telecommunications & Internet Association. Retains the same CTIA initials for which it has been known, and currently presents itself as CTIA–The Wireless Industry.

  Digital wireless users outnumber analog subscribers.

  Wireless subscribers in America exceed 100 million, totaling approximately 38 percent of the U.S. population.

  RESEARCH: Biological risks of ELF continue to receive attention. (Stepansky et al., 2000)

- 2001: FCC votes to raise CMRS (Continuous Monitoring and Risk Scoring) spectrum limits for individual carriers from 45 MHz to 55 MHz, and subsequently eliminates the cap in 2003.

  The average wireless consumer uses his or her phone for 320 minutes per month. (That's 10.6 minutes a day.)

- 2002: Camera phones are first introduced in the U.S. market.

  RESEARCH: Biological effects of EMR on immune function is shown. (Lai, , 2002)

- 2003: The FCC creates a "secondary market" which permits licensees to lease any amount of their spectrum.

  Microsoft introduces Xbox Live, the first Internet-connected gaming hub. At launch, the service is a conduit for downloading additional game content, but it quickly expands to include streaming and video-chat services, including Netflix and Skype.

- 2004: Facebook begins.

  RESEARCH: Extremely Low Frequencies (ELFs) are demonstrated to open the blood-brain barrier, substantiating the earlier work by Frey and others. (IEEE, 2004)

- 2005: Deficit Reduction Act of 2005 enables Digital TV transition and directs the auctioning of 700 MHz of spectrum licenses, raising almost $19 billion for the U.S. Treasury. Money, money, money!

  Wireless subscribers use more than 1.5 trillion voice minutes and send and receive more than 81 billion SMS (Short Message Service) text messages.

  Wireless subscribers reach nearly 208 million, approximately 69 percent of the total U.S. population.

  YouTube launches.

  Google Maps becomes available.

- 2006: Advanced Wireless Services (AWS-1) auction concludes in September and raises nearly $14 billion for the U.S. Treasury. Cha-ching! Cha-ching!

  Google announces in October that it has bought YouTube for $1.65 billion.

  Aircell successfully bids $31.3 million for FCC air-to-ground broadband frequency license.

  Twitter tweets.

- 2007: iPhone launches, dramatic handset innovation.

  RESEARCH: First BioInitiative report is published. It collates nearly 2,000 scientific articles written by scientists around the world, warning of health hazards from EMR. (Sage, 2007)

  Electric utility smart meters begin to be installed in the U.S.

- 2008: iTunes Application Store and Android Play Store open.

There are more than 270 million wireless subscribers who use more than 2.2 trillion minutes; more than 1 trillion text messages, are sent and received in the U.S.

RESEARCH: Cognitive impairment is linked to EMR exposure. (Nittby et al., 2008)

RESEARCH: Another study looked at all the kids who were born in Denmark in a given year and found that mothers who had used mobile phones the most during pregnancy had the greatest risk of having children with behavioral difficulties, including autism and ADHD-like behaviors. The increase in risk was statistically significant. The risk also increased if the child used a cell phone. (Divan et al., 2008)

- 2009: RESEARCH: Further implication of the role of ELF and the permeation of the blood-brain barrier. Scientists demonstrate that low levels of EMF open up the blood-brain barrier. (Eberhardt et al., 2008).

Wireless subscribers use more than 6.2 billion minutes per day and send and receive more than 5 billion text messages per day.

CTIA reports more than 285.6 million U.S. wireless subscriber connections, or approximately 91 percent of the total U.S. population. (Foresman, 2010)

One billionth WiFi chipset is sold.

Palm Software Store, BlackBerry App World, Nokia Ovi Store, Palm App Catalog, and Windows Mobile Marketplace app stores open.

RESEARCH: The immune system is at risk. A study verifies earlier research showing EMR exposure led to cell damage and a reduction in cell tissue repair function. (Johansson, 2009)

- 2010: First 4G handset is introduced at International CTIA Wireless show; FCC proposes National Broadband Plan, recommending 500 MHz of spectrum be allocated for commercial use by 2020.

iPad and other tablets become popular.

Introduction of wireless routers fast and wide-reaching enough to cover the demands of an entire house, coffee shop, or small office from a single access point.

- 2012: RESEARCH: The BioInitiative report is updated and published, listing more than 1,800 additional scientific, peer-reviewed studies on the health hazards of electromagnetic radiation, for a combined total of more than 3,800 studies.

  RESEARCH: Interphone study downplays the risk of cell phone radiation. However, the International Agency for Research on Cancer (IARC) eventually classifies cell phone radiation as a class 2B "Possible Carcinogen." Dr. Joseph Mercola comments on this in his article, "EMF Controversy Exposed."

PAUSE:

The telecommunications industry continues to invent and expand unrelentingly. There is no sign of a slow-down. And why should there be? This is what the world wants. Each year, I attend the CES (Consumer Electronics Show) in Las Vegas and am amazed at the increase in vendors and attendees from all around the globe. (Ironically, the CES actually lost power in 2018 for a few hours during the show.)

Yet, not all are exuberant about this seemingly unstoppable boom. Consortiums of scientific researchers are meeting. Books and blogs are written. Grassroots safety advocacy groups are springing up. Documentary films are produced—all agreeing on the dangers of EMR, or at least agreeing upon its unproven safety claims.

A U.S. Government Accountability Office (GAO) study concludes that "Some consumers may use mobile phones against the body, which FCC does not currently test, and could result in RF energy exposure higher than the FCC limit."

ONWARD:

- 2013: RESEARCH: Study concludes that the regular and long-term use of microwave devices (mobile phone, microwave oven) can have a negative impact upon a biological system, especially on the brain. (Kesari et al., 2013)

  RESEARCH: Another study looks at disease occurrences and proximity to cell towers. (Khurana et al., 2013)

  World Health Organization (WHO) concludes that EMF is a possible human carcinogen.

  The American Cancer Society (ACS) states that the IARC (International Agency for Research on Cancer) classification means that there could be some cancer risk associated with radio-frequency energy, but the evidence is not strong enough to be considered causal and needs to be investigated further.
- 2014: Body-adapted Wearable Electronics and virtual reality become popular.

  RESEARCH: Study implicates EMR to influence a range of bodily functions. Scientists urge attention to more research, given the ubiquitous nature, widespread applications, and capability to produce deleterious effects. (Singh & Kapoor, 2014)
- 2015: Introduction of mobile phone pay systems, drones, smart homes, smart appliances, smart cars, smart watches, virtual reality headsets.

  RESEARCH: The FDA (Food and Drug Administration) nominates the National Toxicology Program (NTP) to study the effects of EMR on health. The NTP raises questions and finds links between EMR and some cancers.
- 2016: The Internet of Things (IoT)—the technologies and standards in the IoT platform provide the basis for

communicating, controlling, managing, and securing endpoints in the IoT. The platforms aggregate data to make the IoT a reality.

Driverless cars, smart homes, more smart devices.

RESEARCH: The National Toxicology Program continues experiments in rats and mice on potential health hazards from cell phone radio-frequency radiation. NTP releases a preliminary report of important findings in May 2016.

- 2017: RESEARCH: Study links risk of miscarriage to electromagnetic field exposure. (De-Kun Li et al., 2017)

  RESEARCH: National Toxicology Program (NTP) completes its research. Results show increased occurrence of rare brain tumors called gliomas in male rats and increases in nerve tumors called schwannoma of the heart, thymus and mediastinum in both male and female rats. (Coldewey, 2018) See Appendix VII for an explanation of the levels of carcinogenicity, as defined by the National Toxicology Program, that are assigned in the results of research studies.
- 2018: In February, NTP held a press conference and said the complete findings conclude that the increases in tumors of nerves in the heart, called malignant schwannomas, were due to the exposures to radiofrequency radiation in male rats. Tumors in the brains were also associated with exposures to cell phone radio-frequency radiation.

  RESEARCH: In March, weighing in on the carcinogenic potential of EMR/EMF, the peer review of the NTP study confirms two categories of "Clear Evidence," three instances of "Some Evidence," and fifteen cases of "Equivocal Evidence." ***There were no parts of this study that showed "No Evidence."*** Results of the NTP study were compiled by Joel M. Moskowitz, PhD, director of the Center for Family and Community

Health at the University of California, Berkeley. See Appendix II for a link to the full transcript of the NTP press conference as well as links to technical reports and experts' analyses of the NTP study.

For up-to-date analyses of the NTP study, here are two excellent sources:

Cellular Phone Task Force: cellphonetaskforce.org
Microwave News: microwavenews.com

- 2019: RESEARCH: As a follow-up, the NTP submitted a manuscript that evaluated DNA damage in three regions of the brain, the liver, and in blood cells in rats and mice. The cells were previously removed during the ongoing two-year toxicology study. NTP scientists found that Radio Frequency Radiation exposure was associated with significant increase in DNA damage. DNA damage, if not repaired, can potentially lead to tumors.

  For NTP updates, go to: ntp.niehs.nih.gov.

He Said, She Said

So, why is there so much contradiction and confusion in the headlines?

Recall, for a moment, the walk down memory lane where we examined things we once thought were safe, but were really not. Remember the smoke and mirrors of the tobacco company? And how the government, news media, medical associations, and the public remained willfully ignorant for a very long time?

Déjà vu all over again.

The cell phone industry pressures our state and federal representatives and regulatory agency officials to enact legislation and implement regulations favorable to the industry. The industry's research findings related to cell phone exposure claim (as the tobacco industry did) there is no conclusive evidence of health risks, and telecommunications industry officials label the people who dispute those claims as fear mongers and conspiracy theorists.

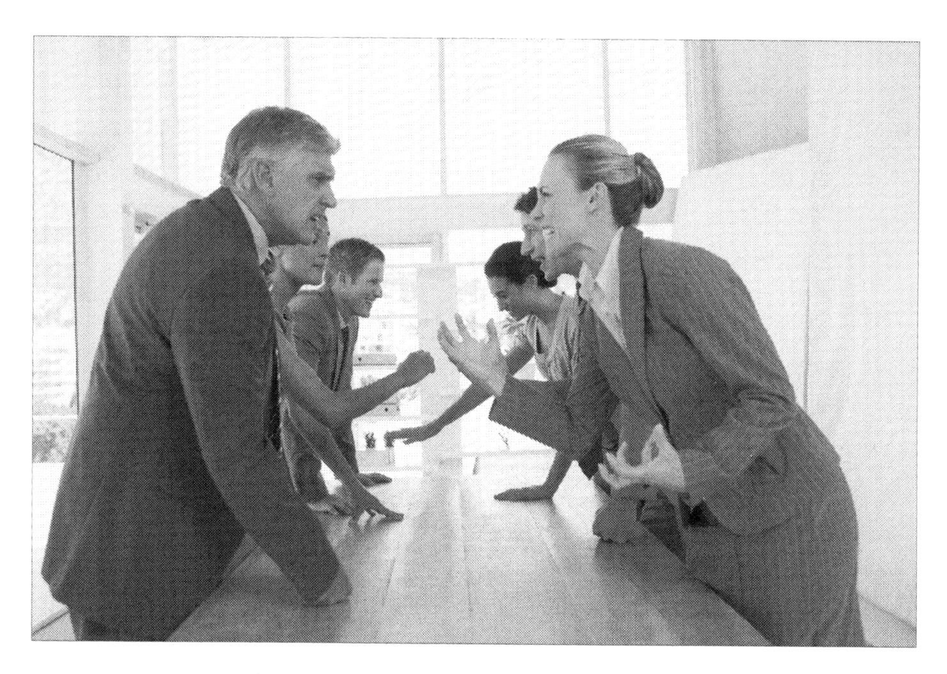

So, what does the research really say and why all this confusion? There are important details in any study that must be meticulously adhered to and transparently reported. There are many ways that scientific mercenaries are able to misrepresent and minimize the truth of good research. They include:

- ✓ Length of study—research can simply be shortened, lacking sufficient duration to achieve results consistent with previous studies.
- ✓ Choice of subjects—lumping participants who rarely use their cell phones at all into a group of "heavy cell phone users," would certainly skew results.
- ✓ The devil is in the details—industry researchers are able to craft studies that are very close to the original, but leave out one important procedural detail, claiming that the results were not able to be replicated.
- ✓ The whole truth and nothing but the truth—research projects can be multifaceted. An announcement may quote a statement from a scientist regarding one small

part of the project that seems to downplay the hazards of EMFs. But the announcement fails to cite subsequent statements of high concern, thus tipping the entire conclusion toward little concern.

✓ Grouping dissimilar diseases together—tt is true that not all kinds of tumors have increased. But some have dramatically increased. One cannot include all types into one number and expect to show an honest result.

✓ Discredit the person—some brilliant and brave scientists have been accused of producing fraudulent findings, only subsequently to have been cleared. Regrettably, the reversal of the accusations are either not reported or buried in a subscript on the back page of something no one reads.

✓ Do it until you get it right—or until you get it wrong. If you repeat an experiment enough times, you will eventually get some ambiguity. It could be because the subjects were compromised in some way. Or some procedure was mishandled. I read about one such experiment that was re-run over and over, until finally, the numbers were such that it could be reported as, "inconclusive." In this particular case, a lot of dogs had to suffer to achieve the "wrong" results.

✓ Realistic Exposure Levels—DDT: Dosage, Distance, Time are all critical factors in determining relevant results.

✓ Source of Funding—an examination of 59 studies on cell phone safety was conducted comparing sources of funding with results and conclusions. Industry-funded studies were least likely to report a statistically significant result that suggested cell phone usage could be hazardous to one's health.

(Huss et al., 2007; Cooper, 2009; Marino, 2010; Morgan, 2011; Davis, 2013; Prasad et al., 2017; Walker, 2017)

In spite of what I call "bureaucratic persecution," good, independent, peer-reviewed, scientific research continues to be published:

A 2017 study of human exposure to non-ionizing radiation from magnetic fields in pregnant women found a significantly higher rate of miscarriage. Researcher Dr. De-Kun Li took measurements of magnetic fields for 913 pregnant women. Miscarriages were nearly three times higher in women who had the most exposure time to non-ionizing, low frequency EMR. This study provides evidence from a human population that magnetic field non-ionizing radiation could have adverse biological impacts on human health.

One of the strengths of this study was that researchers used an objective measuring device and studied a short-term outcome (miscarriage) rather than an outcome that will occur years later, such as cancer or autoimmune diseases. (Li et al., 2017)

A concerning new study links miscarriages to cell phone radiation. How worried should we be? Non-ionizing radiation may have more of a biological effect than we thought. (Belluz, 2018).

Dr. Martin L. Pall, Professor Emeritus of Biochemistry and Basic Medical Sciences, Washington State University, addresses the hazards of EMF exposure from cancer to cardiac issues. He has a bachelor's degree in physics from Johns Hopkins and a PhD in biochemistry and genetics from Caltech. Since about 2000, he's been scouring the medical literature, integrating and drawing parallels between work done by himself and others. He explains:

There is a huge amount of information out here that nobody has the time to integrate, digest and make connections.

Watch Dr. Pall being interviewed by Dr. Mercola: tinyurl.com/ExposedPall.

So, why do we see conflicting reports on the rise (or lack thereof) of brain tumors?

Not all tumors are created equal. Some types of brain cancer show a statistically significant increase and high correlation to EMR exposure. Other types have remained static and show no increase, in spite of exposure to electromagnetic radiation. So, pro-industry research can lump everything together and "claim" there has been little or no increase.

Here's how it goes:

Senior managers at the National Toxicology Program (NTP) released the preliminary results of their cell phone radiation study in May 2016. (USDHHS, 2016) The researchers were so concerned about the elevated rates of two types of cancer among exposed rats, they believed an immediate public alert was warranted. They considered it unwise to wait for the results to wind their way into a journal sometime the following year. Not surprisingly, the NTP report generated worldwide media attention.

There were some startling reactions. Both the American Cancer Society (ACS) and Consumer Reports immediately shelved their long-held, wait-and-see positions. In a statement issued soon after the NTP's press conference, Otis Brawley, the ACS chief medical officer, said the NTP results mark a "paradigm shift in our understanding of radiation and cancer risk." He called the NTP report "good science." Consumer Reports said the new study was "groundbreaking" and encouraged people to take simple precautions to limit their exposures. (Microwave News, 2018)

However, much of the mainstream news media saw it very differently. The *Washington Post* ran its story under the headline, "Do Cell Phones Cause Cancer? Don't Believe the Hype." (Feltman, 2016)

One question on many people's minds was, if cell phones cause cancer, why hasn't there been an increase in the incidence of brain tumors. For example, a reporter at *The New York Times* gave the National Toxicology Program study zero credibility. The reporter said, in a video, that there is "overwhelming evidence" that cell phones do not lead to cancer. "Despite the explosion of cell phone use," the reporter said, "it looks like the incidence of brain cancer has remained pretty much rock steady since 1992." The conclusion was that, "You can use a cell phone without worrying." (Laffin & Kolata, 2016)

Nearly two years later, in February 2018, the NTP itself seemed to downplay its initial findings, stating that upon further review of the data, "it was unclear if the tumors were related to the exposures" of radio-frequency radiation. (USDHHS, 2018)

The *Las Vegas Review Journal* subsequently featured the article, "Hang up on cancer-cell phone link." (AP, 2018)

What, Me Worry?

Question: Are More People Getting Brain Tumors? Or not?

Answer: There's More Than One Type of Brain Tumor

The issue of whether brain tumor rates are static or rising is more complicated than the above articles would have us believe. It's true that the overall incidence of brain tumors has been steady, but a different picture emerges if one carefully examines the data. For example, reported incidences of glioblastoma multiforme (GBM), the most virulent type of brain tumor, ARE rising.

The following graph helps reveal the truth. It's based on brain tumor data from The Netherlands. The black segment of each column tracks the incidence of glioblastoma multiforme. While the total incidence of all types of brain tumors in The Netherlands rose at the rate of only about 0.7 percent per year, the increase in GBM was about 3.1 percent per year. That is, the incidence more than doubled over the period 1989-2010. (Follow the thin line superimposed on the histogram to track the trend.) This is a statistically significant increase. At the same time, the rate of all the other types of brain tumors went down; these changes are also significant. The higher incidence of GBMs is being masked by the lower rates of the other types of brain cancer.

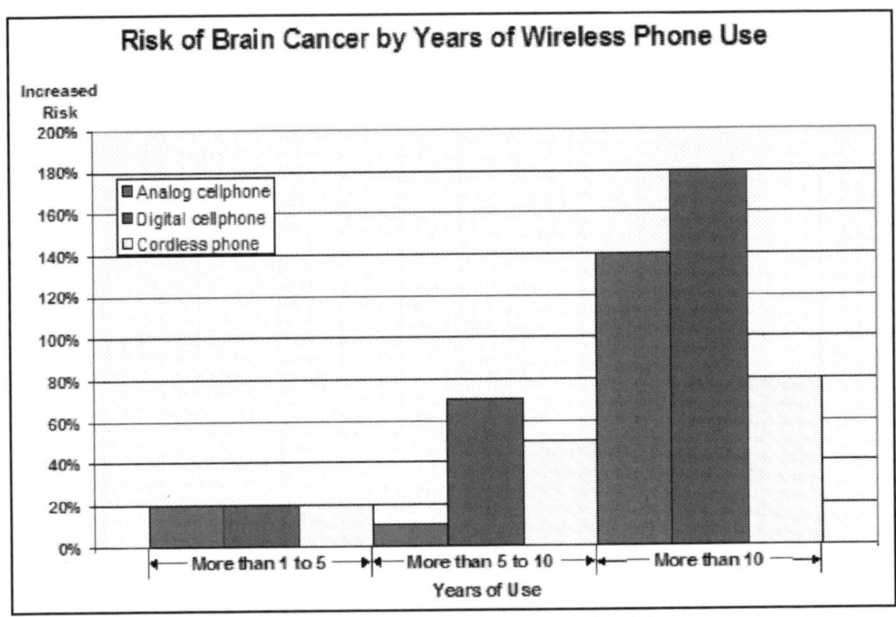

(Morgan, 2006; Hardell et al., 2006) [Reprinted with permission of Lloyd Morgan, PowerWatch.org.]

GBM Tumors Are Rising in the U.S.

A similar trend is occurring in the U.S. Researchers from the University of Southern California looked at the incidence of brain tumors over a 15-year period (1992-2006). In 2012, they published a paper reporting that incidences of GBMs had gone up while the other types had gone down. The study showed "decreased rates of primary brain tumors in all sites with the notable exception of increased incidence of GBM in the frontal lobes, temporal lobes and cerebellum." (Zada et al., 2012)

The increase in GBMs in the temporal lobe (the region of the brain closest to the ear and potentially to a phone) ranged from approximately 1.3 percent to 2.3 percent per year, a finding that is statistically significant. However, the NTP retracted its previous public health warning, saying it's "not a high-risk situation." (Microwave News, 2018; USDHHS, 2018)

Are More People Getting Brain Tumors?
GBMs, the Most Virulent Type, Are Rising

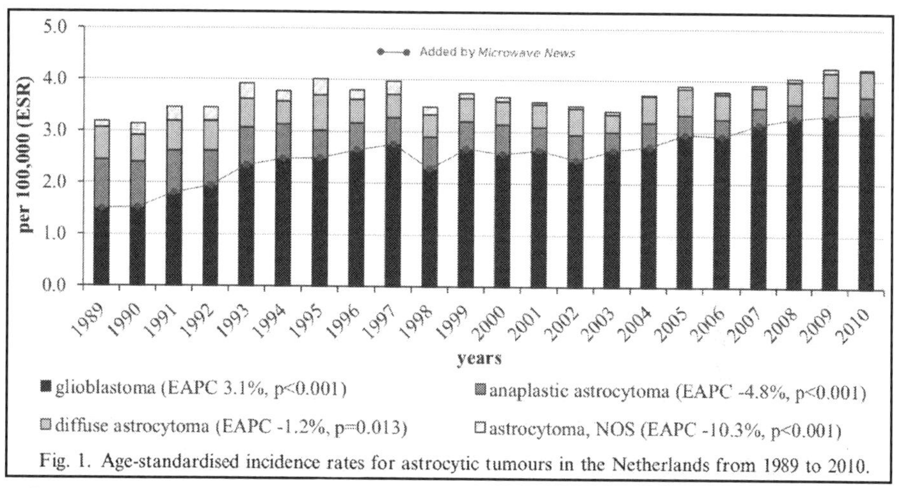

Fig. 1. Age-standardised incidence rates for astrocytic tumours in the Netherlands from 1989 to 2010.

[Source: Adapted from Ho et al., *European Journal of Cancer*, 2014, p.231. Reprinted with permission. The original appears on MicrowaveNews.com at microwavenews.com/news-center/ntp-and-brain-tumor-rates.]

More Contradictions—He Said, She Said

"Power frequency electromagnetic fields and health. Where's the evidence?" That's the title of an article published in the journal *Physics in Medicine & Biology*. (Preece et al., 2000)

If I had not researched this myself, I would have thought I was reading research funded by the tobacco industry. This abstract has almost identical verbiage, claiming:

- No associations have been shown.
- Magnetic fields are not associated with cancer.
- Some epidemiological studies may be interpreted as suggesting a slight increase in the risk of childhood leukemia, possibly from small biases and errors.
- EMR may not be the entire answer.
- Most experts conclude that exposure to EMR is not a human health hazard.

- A possible low risk may be associated.
- There is insufficient evidence to warrant aggressive regulatory concern.
- Further research is needed.

InspectAPedia, a free, Internet-based Encyclopedia of Building & Environmental Inspection, Testing, Diagnosis, Repair, has several articles debunking the "Cancer Scare."

It asks the question, "What does 'Double the Risk of Leukemia Really Mean?'" The conclusion is that the risk is extremely low—much less than the risks posed by a large number of much more common hazards to which people are exposed daily.

And I found this title to be interesting, "Cancer Risk from Lawn Herbicides Is Greater than from Electromagnetic Fields."

A reporter, writing for Vox Media's The Verge, said, "Driving and texting is much more likely to kill you than cell phone radiation. So why are we still talking about the radiation?"

In the article—titled "Cellphone radiation may never stop scaring people, no matter what"—the reporter goes on to quote cancer epidemiologist Geoffrey Kabat as saying, "There's never an 'all clear' sounded for any of these borderline risks out there." (Becker, 2018)

To which I say, Dr. Martin Pall's comment bears repeating:

"There is a huge amount of information out here that nobody has the time to integrate, digest and make connections [between]."

And that's why I wrote this book. It's not always easy to discern between truth and error. Who has the time to plod through the research? And even if the issue proves to be urgently problematic to our health, are there realistic solutions? (Yes. See Section II.)

A review of Chapter 1 will refresh your memory on the research behind three critical health concerns:

Electromagnetic Radiation:

1. Damages DNA.
2. Compromises the Blood-Brain Barrier.
3. Weakens the Immune System.

How are industry safety standards set?

Guidelines on cell phone radiation exposure were set by the FCC, along with input from the Food and Drug Administration (FDA), the Environmental Protection Agency (EPA), the National Institute for Occupational Safety and Health (NIOSH), and the Occupational Safety and Health Administration (OSHA). These standards have not been updated since 1996. Think about that. Where were you and what were you doing in 1996?

Would the automotive industry be allowed to continue following the car safety devices from 1996?

Listed below are some of the main criteria used by the FDA in determining SAR (Specific Absorption Rate) for cell phones in 1996. As you read, ask yourself some pertinent questions, such as:

- How has cell phone use changed since 1996?
- How have the phones themselves evolved since 1996?
- What age groups have adopted cell phone use since 1996?
- What has research shown about cell phone radiation exposure since 1996?

Interestingly, the FCC set the guidelines for cell phones. Yet, the FCC is not responsible for the safety thereof.

Heat: "Safety standards" for cell phones use HEAT transfer into the brain to set safety standards. But research shows that by the time there is measurable heat, the damage has already been done. Safety guidelines for radiation-emitting devices are based on the Specific Absorption Rate, known as the SAR value. The SAR value is a measure of the energy emitted by the cell phone and its potential for heating tissues—but the SAR is only a gauge of the thermal impact of cell phone usage. It has been demonstrated that the non-thermal effects of chronic low-frequency exposure is also biologically damaging. (Volkow et al., 2011; Mercola, 2012)

Exposure times: Would you trust research showing the safety of a cell phone that is used for ***six minutes a day***? Radiation exposure is cumulative and exposure times are important. There are no long-term studies verifying the safety thereof. And remember, SAR levels are severely out-of-date with current consumer usage, by a LOT.

The Age Factor: Young children whose brains and DNA are still developing are much more susceptible to harmful effects of radiation. According to a 2011 Pew Research report, 66 percent of all U.S. children acquire a cell phone before the age of seven, and 87 percent of teens sleep with them under or next to their pillows while connected to the network and emitting microwave radiation into their heads throughout the night. (Sage & Carpenter, 2012; Davis, 2013; Singer, 2014)

The trouble with the cell phone radiation standard is that the standard used by federal regulators may not be the best measure of safety, nor is it the best way to help concerned consumers reduce their exposure. (Reardon, 2011) And remember from Chapter 1 that SAR is based on SAM, which represents a small sample of the total population.

No long-term, human studies, as of yet. But we may get an unintended one in about 15 years. Sigh ...

One analysis projected a very large increase in brain cancer incidence beginning in approximately 10 years resulting from widespread mobile phone use. This projection was based on well-established effects of cell phone radiation on DNA mutations, along with the finding that mobile phone use decreases the efficiency of the repair of mutated DNA.

Lloyd Morgan, an electronics engineer and board member of the Central Brain Tumor Registry of the United States warns, "What this analysis shows is that, unless mobile phone usage behavior patterns significantly change, we can reasonably expect a pandemic of brain tumors, for which we are ill-prepared."

"Governments, as well as parents, physicians, schools, and all citizens, would be well advised to educate all persons under their care or influence about the need to curtail the use of mobile phones and other radiation-emitting consumer devices." (Mercola, 2012)

Who is looking out for our health concerns?

Let's Engage in Some Skepticism

You may have heard the claims from industry and government spokespersons that the majority of studies show that wireless phones do not pose a health risk.

I am telling you that is not true.

When industry-funded research is removed, the overwhelming weight of evidence shows that there IS a significant correlation between EMR/EMF exposure and disease. Which of the 5,000 studies do you not believe?

You may have read that brain tumors have decreased, not increased, as one would expect if cell phones were a factor in brain cancer.

Yet, I have read that some types of brain tumors have increased significantly. Interestingly, they are the tumors closest to where a cell phone is usually positioned. Additionally, some tumors have a long latency period. The fact that some have decreased doesn't make me feel any safer. I'm not willing to "wait and see" on this one.

You say, cell phones meet the FCC safety standards and that's good enough for me.

To that, I reply, "reeeeelly?" Those standards were set in 1996, using SAM, and tissue heating as the test. What was your cell phone usage in 1996 and how strong was your phone, if you even had one. Research shows biological changes from ELFs (extremely low frequencies). And those ELFs are about a thousand times lower than the FCC limits. I'd rather trust an ELF than the government. (Take another walk down Memory Lane.)

Consumers for Safe Phones published the article "Exposing the Industry's Lies About Cell Phone Radiation." It is worth reading; see Appendix VI. *BioInitiative 2012* also addresses this issue. (Hardell et al., 2012).

Now, back to your objections. You allow your children to use digital devices, but only for a couple hours a day. It must be safe, or we would all know about it. And WiFi is used in schools. They wouldn't allow that if it were not safe.

My answer? Children's brains absorb 50 to 75 percent more microwave radiation from cell phones than do adult brains. Their delicate DNA is still developing. The FCC did not address children and pregnant women in its tests, unless SAM can somehow represent a seven-year-old or a baby in the womb. Besides, wired technology costs more. So, WiFi is better on the school budget.

You may argue that the World Health Organization (WHO), National Cancer Institute, and American Cancer Society would all be screaming an alarm if there were any danger in wireless usage.

To which I answer: Read.

In 2011, the WHO classified cell phone radiation exposure as a Class 2B carcinogen, placing it in the same health risk category as lead and DDT. The National Cancer Institute's website states, "More research is needed because cell phone technology and how people use cell phones have been changing rapidly." And, from the American Cancer Society's website, "It is important that the possible risk of cell phone exposure continue to be researched using strong study methods, especially with regard to use by children and longer term use."

You might appeal to the really smart people in the ICNIRP (International Commission on Non-Ionizing Radiation Protection) and the IEEE (Institute of Electrical and Electronics Engineers). These groups should be able to give a definitive answer to this question, but the public has not been issued any serious warning from them.

From what I can glean, the ICNIRP uses "heating" as its threshold, which is waaaay past the point of cellular damage. Their position in the past has been, basically, "no heat, no danger." And it may have some ties to industry, as well. As for IEEE, engineers tend to study the physical properties of electricity, formulas and equations rather than biological effects at the cellular level. While these people are very smart and do add valuable research, they do not represent the complete picture when it comes to the biological effects of EMR/EMF.

I hear you grasping at one last straw: What about all the inconsistencies? Even like-minded, independent scientists admit to differences in results. And here's one for you: The NTP reports that in one segment of that study, several of the exposed rats out-lived the control group.

Life. That's my answer. What do I mean by that? Unlike gravity and other physical laws, which exact 100 percent compliance from 100 percent of its subjects, 100 percent of the time, biological research involving living creatures does not guarantee uniform response to a stimulus.

This can be verified by simple observation and common sense. Living beings have unsearchable, complex variables of genetics, immunity, personality, etc. Consequently, it is impossible to have an identical, one-to-one correspondence between subjects exposed to a stimulus and those in a control group. This is why everyone exposed to an infectious disease will not contract that disease, and why everyone who takes the same medicine will not achieve the expected results, and why all of the little rodents will not die according to a predictable time chart. Life is more than spinning electrons and electrical-chemical impulses. It cannot be contained in an exact formula or equation.

The fact that contradictions exist in no way diminishes the patterns of evidence and the volumes of statistically significant data demonstrating that EMFs have a negative effect on the health of living creatures. That's life.

Final Arguments

You tell me that you are healthy. You just don't buy all the hype. You are not the least bit afraid. You just don't have a sense of urgency about this. There are millions of users who have no health issues at all.

I guess you could also assert that there were plenty of smokers who did not get lung cancer. And that there were non-smokers who did come down with lung cancer. Would that free you to safely light a cigarette?

You could also argue that there are people who do not apply sun screen and do not wear sunglasses. They do not all get skin cancer or eye damage. But does that make you feel safe to not protect yourself from sun damage?

Additionally, most people don't get serious injuries in an auto accident. But does that mean that you would not wear a seatbelt? Or would you feel safe having the airbags disabled?

Suppose everything I have written in this book is wrong. Or, pretend that in all 67,000 words in this book, only half of them are correct. Even so, what would be the harm in implementing the solutions in Section II?

What's it going to cost you?

✓ A few minutes of forethought.
✓ Relocating some of your electronics.
✓ Adopting some new habits.
✓ And possibly a small amount of money.

Or, suppose that half of more than 5,000 studies (so far) implicating EMR/EMFs as dangerous to health and well-being are mistaken. So, what if only 2,500 are valid? Or, what if only 1,250 of the research projects compellingly demonstrated that EMR/EMFs were hazardous to our health? And what if only 625 studies actually drew the correct conclusions that this is a serious impact on our health? Didn't the conclusion that smoking was hazardous to health start with one research study in 1929? How many studies would be necessary to convince you?

So, what if the position of this book, and others like it, is correct. What if there IS something to this?

Are you willing to risk your health and the health of the people you love by waiting until the government and news media get on board and reveal the dangers of this? It took decades for the truth about smoking and other elements of harm to be admitted by those in positions of authority and influence. But the voices of truth were sounding out loud and clear well before that. Will you pay attention to the "Watchmen on the Wall?"

As long as the jury is still out on this—similar to the jury being hung up for so many decades on the dangers of smoking and other harmful substances that we once thought were safe—I think we could all stand to change our habits, "just in case." Just as we put on sun screen to reduce the risk of skin cancer, and wear sun glasses to reduce the risk of eye damage, and we take preventive measures to reduce the risk of a heart attack.

To whom will you entrust your health and the health of your children and pets?

Studies have shown:

- "Smoking is safe."
- "OxyContin is non-addicting."
- "Wonder Bread builds bodies 12 ways."
- "Go ahead, drink the Kool-Aid."

Ovem lupo commitere = To entrust a wolf to guard sheep.

Actions for Today:

✓ Research the research.
✓ Don't rely on industry, governmental agencies, or the news media to keep you safe.
✓ Take charge of your own health today.

Need or want solutions right now?

Go to Chapters 7, 8 and 9 (more than 30 pages of solutions) and Appendix I for your Comprehensive Home Safety Audit.

Chapter 4

What's Smart?

Dirty Diapers, the "Creepy Line," and Other Emerging Technologies

Diapers: Time for a Change

Smart diapers now send a signal to the parent (or nanny) that the diaper is wet. Yes! I'm not kidding. Like the baby monitor, radiation is being emitted directly at the baby, and also to the recipient of the message. Like the baby monitor, you must measure it to ensure safety. But unlike the baby monitor, which can be moved away to create some distance from the source, the diaper, by its very nature, must be wrapped around the baby's abdomen. No getting around that. (Freeman, 2014)

Google: The "Creepy Line"

When Eric Schmidt, former executive chairman of Google, was interviewed regarding the technology giant's reach into our personal data, email, passwords, and search history, he made some disturbing statements.

"We don't need you to type at all because we know where you are (with your permission). We know where you've been (with your permission). We can more or less guess what you're thinking about."

"There's what I call the 'Creepy Line,' and the Google policy about a lot of these things is to get right up to the 'Creepy Line' but not cross it."

"I would agree that implanting something in your brain is the 'Creepy Line,' at least until the technology gets better."

Think about that. Do technological advances influence what is or is not ethical? Sounds creepy to me. (Sol, 2014)

Smart Glasses and Beyond

There are smart glasses that are currently being used. And then there is the next evolution that is being released. These new smart glasses actually project "VCSELs" (vertical-cavity surface-emitting lasers) directly onto your retina. Check out this awesome seven-minute video, "Intel's New Smart Glasses Hands On": youtube/bnfwClgheF0.

Are they safe? "Absolutely!"

Thermo "Safer" Smart Monitoring Body Thermometer

Affix a silicone patch to your baby. A wireless sensor will sound an alarm if your baby's temperature is abnormal. It will even produce a graph. No need to touch your little tyke. Just trust the technology. It even won an award for baby technology.

Microchip: Wave Bye-Bye

As of August 2017, employees at Three Square Market, a technology company in Wisconsin, can choose to have a chip the size of a grain of rice injected between their thumb and index finger. Once that is done, any task involving Radio Frequency Identification (RFID) technology—swiping into the office building, paying for food in the cafeteria—could be accomplished with a wave of the hand. (BBC News, 2017)

The program is not mandatory, but as of the following Monday, more than 50 out of 80 employees at Three Square's headquarters in River Falls, Wis., had already signed up.

So, wave bye-bye to any chance of being free from constant WiFi exposure at work, not to mention a host of other issues. Isn't there a movie about this?

Smart Wallets

The smart wallet also has impressive features that will make it very hard to misplace, thanks to two features—a Bluetooth alarm system that will notify the owners every time they leave their wallet behind, and a built-in global GPS system that can track the wallet anywhere in the world in real-time. Additionally, its connectivity systems ensure that the owners will get notifications when they forget their phone behind, and a push button on the wallet that will make your phone ring, even when it's on silent mode. (Waseem, 2017)

Smart House

It's the cool thing—just speak, and it will be done. Let there be light—lights on. TV off. Play my favorite song. It's a wonderful life. The Jetsons! And all that data is stored . . . where?

The number of smart home products—devices that let you control your lighting, thermostat, or even your crock pot and coffee maker from your smartphone—continues to grow. Tons of products and whole ecosystems want to help you control your home via a single touch of your phone. (Higginbotham, 2017; Prospero, 2018)

Wireless Charging

WyTricity—wireless charging over radiofrequencies.

Get rid of all wires. You heard me. Cables and cords are on their way out. That's smart!

RF charging over large areas: laptops, phones, tablets, wireless earbuds, you name it. If it has a battery, it can be charged via RF. This one technology, if it delivers the potential that it has, will effectively change the way we live our lives. Manufacturers are developing this for automobiles, homes, and businesses.

Imagine having your phone and laptop automatically charged, just by walking into a building. How convenient.

And SPEED like you've never experienced. (Mearian, 2017; Patel, 2017)

Back to the Future Smart Hotel

Staying at a hotel will never be the same.

Fixed-mobile Convergence will offer automatic phone pairing with a guest's room phone. The staff will be able to reach out to a guest regardless of the guest's location. Calls can be forwarded and seamlessly transferred from Wireless to 4G or 5G.

Location Analytics will enable the staff to locate a guest who has placed a dinner order and decided to go to the pool. With location analytics, the staff will easily be able to locate the guest and provide better customer service. And we all want to be served just a little bit faster.

Smart hospitality will know the guests at hotels and engage with them after obtaining powerful knowledge of what they want and when they want it. (LeFebvre, 2017; Paul, 2017)

Mobile Device as Door Key

No need for reassigning room keys. Synchronize guest phones with the proper code through a digital reader, and the worry of lost keys or reprogramming can become a thing of the past. This, combined with location analytics, can make check-in and check-out almost a thing of the past. Quick and Cool! (Siat, 2017)

The Internet of Things (IoT): Be Smart. Be connected.

Some of the IoT products currently being manufactured include driverless cars, WiFi clothing, toasters, coffee makers; even diapers, and pacifiers for babies will be made "smart." There will be "smart" mattresses (with "infidelity detection systems"), "smart" toothbrushes to record and notify you how well you are brushing your teeth, WiFi connected pills to transmit data to your physician, Babypod Bluetooth tampon speaker, an intravaginal speaker that plays music directly to the fetus. (Pallister, 2015; Macdonald, 2016; Stern, 2016; Gazdecki, [Undated])

At the 2020 Consumer Electronics Show (CES) in my home town of Las Vegas, I could not believe all the "smart" inventions that were being marketed! Everything was about being "smart" and "connected."

Does this imply that if you are not buying and using their techno-products that you are dumb and disconnected? Here are a few more Smart devices that I recently saw at CES:

- Smart baby socks: Track your baby's heart rate and oxygen level. (But no mention of measuring sock odor.)
- Smart baby bottle: Keeps track of milk temperature, feeding amount, proper bottle angle, etc. (What happened to the burp?)
- Pump it up: Bluetooth breast pump for nursing mothers. Allows mom to multi-task.
- Smart stethoscope: Expectant mothers can check on fetal movement, heart rate, and uterine contraction. 24/7!
- Smart shoe insert: Keeps foot warm, (I like that), and tracks steps and calories. Like the old pedometer. But smarter.
- Smart sleep pillow companion: Improves your sleep via breathing regulation, sounds and snuggling.
- Smart womb: Fetus camera enables you to see your baby's first smile, before he or she makes the grand entrance with a cry.
- Smart footwear: Track your movements and create a custom LED light show activated by your own fancy footwork.
- Smart underwear: Monitors heart rate, breathing, hydration, body fat, temperature, perspiration and lets you know when you're stressed.
- Smart fertility tracker: Tracks temperature and predicts ovulation. Maybe rings a bell when it's time?

- Smart bike helmet: Basically puts your phone function into the helmet. Right up against your head. Includes tail lights and turn signals on the back of the helmet – probably too small to catch the attention of a distracted driver. My wife is a dedicated cyclist. She is not planning on buying this EMR HELLmet.
- Smart pet assistant: Tracks food and water consumption. (I think I'll stick with my cat's meOW.)
- Giddy-UP: The smart saddle will measure the locomotion, power, and heart rate of your horse.
- Ride 'em, cowboy: It's the horseback riders' equivalent to, "I have fallen and I can't get up." Tracks you when you fall and does some analytics on your condition. Ouch!

  I'm not makin' this stuff up—it's the latest, greatest, and smartest from CES.
- Missing Puppy: They've been microchipping pets for years. The difference is that the connecting device remains OFF until the pet goes missing. Then it is activated. It is a passive device that requires no internal power source. The scanning process activates the ID information. Your puppy is safe with us. (PetFinder.com, [Undated])

  (See Appendix I for a comprehensive list of devices.)

5G—"It's a Matter of National Security!"

Seriously! That's the headline to which I recently woke up. It appeared, unsolicited, on my phone. (Google must know that I am tracking this topic.)

The White House had released its annual National Security Strategy report in December 2017. On page 19, in a section on improving America's infrastructure, was this action item: "We will improve America's digital infrastructure by deploying a secure 5G Internet capability nationwide." Other than natural gas, 5G wireless service was the only area of technology to get a specific mention for infrastructure. (Trump, 2017)

But one line in particular tickled the ear of the telecommunications industry:

"We will improve America's digital infrastructure by deploying a secure 5G Internet capability nationwide," the administration wrote. "These improvements will increase national competitiveness, benefit the environment, and improve our quality of life."

Wireless industry group CTIA said that in order to beat rival nations in the race to 5G, the government would need to open up additional spectrum and ease infrastructure regulations.

"CTIA and the wireless industry are pleased that the President's national security strategy acknowledges the critical importance of next-generation 5G wireless to maintaining America's competitiveness," CTIA President and CEO Meredith Attwell Baker said in a statement. (Szal, December 12, 2017)

It's true. It IS a matter of national security to keep up with and be competitive in the digital age. The pro-industry legislation is predictable and unstoppable. The race is ON. (Crichton, 2017)

The cell phone industry is installing upwards of two million small cells on lamp posts, buildings, and power poles in America as part of the ramping up to 5G and IoT. They've got us covered. (Senum, 2017)

But what will this mean for our health?

What's the Matter with 5G, Smart Devices, and IoT?

To review, 5G is one of the most insidious invasions of privacy ever promoted, and until just recently, it was being implemented "under the radar." It can include a type of microwave frequency called millimeter waves (MMW). It's not entirely new. MMWs have been used in medicine and airport security. But it is new for wide-spread continuous general public consumption—and continuous general public exposure.

These millimeter waves are the fastest, shortest, highest-intensity wave lengths within the microwave spectrum.

This is not just an upgrade of 4G. This is the next major evolution in wireless communication. 5G is the central platform for connecting everything to everyone at all times. It will be the necessary technological support for IoT (The Internet of Things).

Here are some of the crucial elements to implementing 5G:

- Density. Network density (i.e., adding more base stations and access points) will be necessary to get network access closer to individual users—along city streets, in buildings, and everywhere in between. That means adding more antennas and small cell sites. Cell towers can now be as close as 250 feet, or one every three to twelve homes in urban or suburban areas, mounted on lampposts. Speeds will be over 20 times faster than the current 4G technology.
- Virtualization. To effectively manage the spectrum, physical equipment will shift to virtualized environments operating in centralized data centers using solutions such as centralized radio access networks (C-RAN), network function virtualization (NFV), and cell virtualization.
- Aggregation: Carrier aggregation combines multiple component carriers across the available spectrum to combine chunks of bandwidth, increase data rates, and improve network performance.
- Massive Multiple Input/Multiple Output (MIMO): Thousands of active antenna elements will work together to provide MIMO.
- Your Smartphone as a Smart HUB: The super high-speed mobile broadband access and truly ubiquitous, laser-sharp coverage will let all of your smart devices communicate directly to one another and your 5G smartphone will act as the Hub. Think of your smartphone as the ultimate universal remote.
- Low Latency: No wait-time for video streaming. Very high reliability, global coverage.

(Miller, 2017)

Once again, there are:

- No pre-market studies.
- No long-term studies.
- No opportunity for an individual to opt-out of this technology.
- It will be EV-ery-where.

IoT, The Internet of Things, is a vast, worldwide computer network linking smaller computer networks.

5G + IoT = $$$ and POW-UH!

There are three defining elements:

1. There is a physical object or device.
2. It is "smart"; i.e., that object is embedded with sensors, microchips, software, and an operating system, and it may include data storage.
3. It uses wireless technology to connect with other devices.

There are lots of smart devices in place right now. What is different about 5G working together with IoT is that the devices will be able to collect and analyze data, communicate with other devices, and automatically perform intelligent actions.

It's not just about having an array of wireless gadgets. It's about connecting them all in a way that serves you better. And don't we have that innate nature that wants to be served?

Here's how it looks:

Sensors collect data about you and your family to determine what's "normal," for you. To serve you better. To make your life easier.

Your smart house knows your habits, how quickly or slowly you move, how many people are normally in your house, what you are doing, when you eat, how many times you get up in the night, how many people normally come and go during a 24-hour period, so that if something out-of-the-ordinary happens, it can alert you. Or alert someone else.

Instead of you programming your coffee maker to start at a certain time, your smart bed lets your smart coffee maker know when you get up. Aaahh, the smell of coffee greets you.

Your smart refrigerator is on the blink. Before you even know it, before you can smell the coffee awaiting you, it has already scheduled a repair technician for a day and time it knows you are available. And diagnostics have been sent ahead and the part has been ordered.

Smart clothing on your toddler can alert you when he or she runs a fever at daycare, or throws a tantrum. You can talk him or her down off that tantrum via your phone. Or, at least you can try.

And your fitness coach gets a detailed report of all your physical activity every day. So there's no fudging on your workouts.

Your smart car communicates with your smart house so that when you are near, it automatically turns on the heat (or air conditioning) and the lights. It can have your favorite music playing when you walk in the door. "Honey, I'm ho-ome." (Miller, 2017)

Let's review and reflect. The IoT knows your comings and your goings, when you come in, when you go out. How many people are in your home. How fast you all move and breathe. So, it could be extraordinarily useful for crime control and national security, busting drug houses and terrorist cells . . . and rooting out young girls (remember Anne Frank?) . . . and there would be no place to hide.

Sigh.

Even if one were to choose not to employ "smart living" devices, the sensors are still with us. And most of your neighbors' homes would presumably be "smart." I can see the privacy issues getting out of hand, not to mention the inescapable EMR exposure stacking up like the Tower of Babel. How much is too much? This much!

While technological advancements can be convenient, and sometimes exhilarating, they also should give one a heightened level of concern about:

- Super-dose, ubiquitous exposure to EMR, 24/7, everywhere you go. Exposure levels even worse than we are already getting.
- What this could potentially do to our initiative and independence? How much is too much?
- Privacy lost, almost to the point of extinction. This is Big Brother on steroids.

It's Coming. It's Already Here. It's Not Going Away.

The Winter Olympics in South Korea are said to be the most high-tech Olympics ever. Major telecom companies showed off their capabilities, such as virtual-reality viewing stations and super-fast video streaming.

"Viewers can control the time, target, even the angle of what they're viewing," said Michelle Toh, a correspondent for CNN. Using 5G, the wireless network technology that mobile carriers around the world have been racing to adopt, Pyeongchang emerged as a testing ground for new technology.

Yes, the race is on, in more ways than one.

What is in the works? AT&T began implementing 5G in Dallas, Atlanta, and Waco, Texas, in 2018. And T-Mobile began building out its 5G network, with plans to be in 30 cities by the end of 2018, including New York, Los Angeles, Dallas, and Las Vegas. (Reichert, 2018; Kastrenakes, 2018)

Can 5G be delayed? Some have tried. In September 2017, more than 180 scientists and doctors from 36 countries appealed to the EU for a 5G moratorium, warning of the potential serious health effects of 5G. They asked for a full investigation of the potential health effects of 5G, independent from industry, asserting that: "5G will substantially increase exposure to radio frequency electromagnetic fields (RF-EMF) on top of the 2G, 3G, 4G, WiFi, etc. for telecommunications already in place. RF-EMF has been proven to be harmful for humans and the environment." (See Appendix IV for the complete statement.)

Furthermore, a statement from the International EMF Alliance urgently called for "a complete overhaul of EMF exposure guidelines based on up-to-date credible information from empirically based life sciences."

However, Joel Moskowitz noted that in its October 2017 response to the 5G Appeal, "the European Commission claims that current limits on RF-EMF exposure established by the International Commission on Non-Ionizing Radiation Protection are adequate to protect the population, and that these limits apply to the frequencies to be deployed for 5G."

Thus, the appeal fell on deaf ears and the 5G rollout in Europe began.

Meanwhile, a groundswell of grassroots efforts contributed to the delay of the implementation of 5G in California in the fall of 2017. A Band-Aid on arterial bleeding, as it turns out. (Moskowitz, August 2017; Szal, 2017)

Can grassroots effort of health advocates bring about a delay long enough to make a difference in the way and speed with which technology advances? Wouldn't it be awesome for U.S. inventors and innovators to engage in a different "race"? A race for safer technology, effective personal shielding, or cloaking mechanisms for homes, or even a pathway to 5G "opt out"? Such a delay would be an opportunity for innovation and a dream win for the U.S.

1. A win for our health.
2. A win for our privacy and freedom.
3. A win in financial success for innovators and inventors.

You see, I am neither anti-technology nor anti-profit. But just not at the expense of my health and privacy.

Ah . . . back to reality.

The CTIA has on its website the following statement:

It's important the United States do everything we can to maintain our wireless leadership. Because when we win the race to 5G, we all win.

Actions for Today:

- ✓ Pause. Determine to keep your life simple and manageable.
- ✓ Retain your plug-in cords and hard wire your electronics when possible.
- ✓ Resist the sensors and listen to your body, soul, and spirit.
- ✓ Make it a point to employ human touch, not techno-touch.
- ✓ Consider joining a local safety advocacy group.
- ✓ And resist the urge to be "cutting edge." It may hurt you.

Need or want solutions right now?

Go to Chapters 7, 8 and 9 (more than 30 pages of solutions) and Appendix I for your Comprehensive Home Safety Audit.

Chapter 5

Why Isn't Everyone Sounding the Alarm?

Why Don't I Hear More About This?

Seven Reasons:

1. Cell Phone Companies
2. WiFi Providers
3. Utility Companies and "Smart Meters"
4. Manufacturers of Electronic Devices
5. Government
6. Consumers
7. Money, Money, Money

If you read the previous chapters carefully, you have some idea of the tremendous power and money behind the telecommunications industry. It is a soon-to-be trillion-dollar industry in the U.S. And the potential for power and profit is incalculable. It is not to the industry's advantage to entertain the idea that there could be any health risks. And when the lawyers get involved, it hinders free-thinking, unbiased research and media reporting. There is often a great deal of intimidation to suppress the truth.

It is the industry's job to create DOUBT about any claims that the technology is unsafe. The following are quotes from "industry experts," from asbestos to tobacco, and now from the telecommunications industries, doing what they do best—creating doubt that there is anything unsafe about their products.

"More research is needed."

"There is no conclusive evidence."

"Many scientists and leading experts disagree."

"Lack of consistent evidence."

"The origin of this disease is shrouded in mystery."

"There is inadequate evidence."

"There is a tremendous tendency to oversimplify."

"Many complex questions remain to be answered."

"We do not know."

"We have a great deal to learn."

"Far too many people rush to a premature judgment."

"Many highly respected members of the scientific community took vigorous exception to the study."

"There are large numbers of us who have some background in this field who do not believe the evidence is sufficient."

"The science is still evolving."

Undoubtedly, the tremendous money and power influence the governmental agencies that are there to protect us, and delay and cloud public communication.

Notice the heavily muted sound-off in the controversial California Department of Public Health report on EMF released, under threat of litigation, by the Division of Environmental and Occupational Disease Control in December 2017. It is reprinted in the sidebar beginning on page 106, with my responses on the facing pages. Can you pick up on the familiar language of DOUBT embedded in the statement?

This statement was never meant to go public; it was officially classified as a "draft." The public release of the guidelines came about in part because University of California researcher Joel Moskowitz, PhD, had sued the state for not making it public.

A superior court judge ruled that the "document advising the public of the risks associated with cellular phones" is not a draft. She ordered the state to release an unaltered version of the public record without the text that it added indicating the document was a "Draft and Not for Public Release."

The document is dated April 2014, but Moskowitz says the document was originally prepared in 2007 and updated several times, but never released to the public. (Albarazi, 2017)

Stop and think about that. These safety guidelines were never meant to be released to the public. And it took the threat of a lawsuit to provide this information.

It does contain some valuable tips, which I include in Section II. However, there are gaping holes in the understanding of this issue. Some of the recommendations don't go nearly far enough. And some assertions are just plain incorrect. Because of that, there may be a false sense of security or safety in some of the short-sighted tips. I would not want to stake my health upon this report. It is a start. But there is so much more that goes unaddressed.

This statement was never meant to go public; it was officially classified as a "draft." The public release of the guidelines came about in part because University of California researcher Joel Moskowitz, PhD, had sued the state for not making it public.

It is reminiscent of the language the tobacco industry used when they realized that health concerns were becoming public. Their approach became: We do not believe there is any cause for alarm . . . but just in case, we've added a new filter to provide safe, worry-free smoking. (Remember, it was an asbestos filter.) And the government cooperated, until it could no longer maintain its complicity. Why should we expect anything different with EMR?

continued on page 116

This statement on EMF was released, under threat of litigation, in December 2017.

Division of Environmental and Occupational Disease Control California Department of Public Health

How to Reduce Exposure to Radiofrequency Energy from Cell Phones

December 22, 2017

The use of cell phones has increased dramatically in recent years, including among children and young adults. These phones put out radio frequency (RF) energy.

Some scientists and public health officials believe RF energy may affect human health. This guidance document describes RF energy, lists some of the potential health concerns, and provides guidance on how people can reduce their exposure.

Why are people concerned about exposure to RF energy from cell phones?

Although the science is still evolving, some laboratory experiments and human health studies have suggested the possibility that long-term, high use of cell phones may be linked to certain types of cancer and other health effects, including:

- brain cancer and tumors of the acoustic nerve (needed for hearing and maintaining balance) and salivary glands
- lower sperm counts and inactive or less mobile sperm
- headaches and effects on learning and memory, hearing, behavior, and sleep

The Truth Is . . .

Does RF energy affect human health?

- Many scientists and public health officials believe RF energy *DOES* affect human health, not "may" affect human health.

Why are people concerned about exposure to RF energy from cell phones?

- Many studies have suggested a strong correlation between cancer and other health effects and EMR/ EMF exposure.

continued from page 108

California Department of Public Health

These studies do not establish the link definitely, however, and scientists disagree about whether cell phones cause these health problems and how great the risks might be.

This document is intended to provide guidance for those people who want to reduce their own and their families' exposures to RF energy from cell phones, despite this uncertainty.

What is RF energy?

Cell phones work by sending and receiving signals to and from cell phone towers. These signals are a form of electromagnetic radiation called radio frequency (RF) energy. Other sources of RF energy include cell phone towers, TV and radio transmitters, smart meters, and microwave ovens. When a phone sends signals to a tower, the RF energy goes from the phone's antenna out in all directions, including into the head and body of the person using the phone. Cell phones also emit RF energy when using WiFi and/or Bluetooth, but at lower levels. RF energy is not as powerful or as damaging to cells or DNA as some other kinds of electromagnetic radiation, such as X-rays or UV rays from the sun. Some scientific studies have, however, suggested that there may be increased health risks from exposure to RF energy.

How can you reduce your exposure?

- Keep your phone away from your body. Keeping your phone just a few feet away from you can make a big difference.

  When you talk on your cell phone, avoid holding it to your head—use the speakerphone or a headset

continued from page 109

The Truth Is . . .

- There are thousands of studies that do establish a statistically significant, dose-related correlation between EMR/EMF exposure and disease.
- The majority of scientists who are not funded by industry do agree that this poses a serious health hazard, or at least that its safety is unproven.

What is RF energy?

- Accurate in terms of the technology. However, many scientists and public health officials believe exposure to RF energy *DOES* increase health risks, not "may" increase health risks.

How can you reduce your exposure?

- True. Across the room is even better.
- Yes, use speaker phone. Wired headsets might be OK, but they must be measured to be sure. Where are you carrying your phone when using a headset? As for wireless Bluetooth headsets, I've never measured one

continued from page 110

California Department of Public Health

instead. Wireless (Bluetooth) and wired headsets emit much less RF energy than cell phones.

- Send text messages instead of talking on the phone.
- If you are streaming or if you are downloading or sending large files, try to keep the phone away from your head and body.
- Carry your cell phone in a backpack, briefcase, or purse, NOT in a pocket, bra or belt holster. Because your phone's antenna tries to stay connected with a cell tower whenever it's on, it emits some RF energy even when you are not using it. It does not emit RF energy when it's in airplane mode. (Airplane mode turns off cellular, WiFi, and Bluetooth.)

Reduce or avoid using your cell phone when it is sending out high levels of RF energy. This happens mainly when:

- You see only one or two bars displayed. Cell phones put out more RF energy to connect with cell towers when the signal is weak. If you must use your phone when the signal is weak, try to follow the other guidance on this page.
- You are in a fast-moving car, bus, or train. Your phone puts out more RF energy to maintain connections to avoid dropping calls as it switches from one cell tower to the next unless it is in airplane mode.
- You are streaming audio or video, or downloading or sending large files. To watch movies or listen to playlists on your phone, download them first, then switch to airplane mode while you watch or listen.

continued from page 111

The Truth Is . . .

that was in the safe range. My meters indicate that bursts of radiation occur every 6-30 seconds on the average.

- Texting: Yes, but consider where you are you holding your phone when you text.
- Where to carry the device: First, a purse or backpack is not far enough away to decrease radiation danger. Second, not all phones automatically turn off all radiation with airplane mode. Some do, some don't. You need to double check and make sure WiFi and Bluetooth are also off. And re-check periodically, as some phones can turn WiFi and Bluetooth features back on, even when you are in airplane mode.

Reduce or avoid using your cell phone when it is sending out high levels of RF energy.

- Low bars: Unless there is an emergency, wait until your reception is optimal.

- Fast-moving vehicle: True, but double check to make sure that airplane mode is ON, and WiFi and Bluetooth are OFF.

- Streaming or downloading: Better yet, as far away as possible.
- Viewing: Make sure Bluetooth and WiFi are off.

continued from page 112

California Department of Public Health

Don't sleep with your phone in your bed or near your head.

Unless the phone is off or in airplane mode, keep it at least a few feet away from your bed.

Take off the headset when you're not on a call.

Headsets release small amounts of RF energy even when you are not using your phone.

Don't rely on a "radiation shield" or other products claiming to block RF energy, electromagnetic fields, or radiation from cell phones.

According to the U.S. Federal Trade Commission, products that interfere with the phone's signal may force it to work harder and emit more RF energy in order to stay connected, possibly increasing your exposure.

What about children?

Children may be more at risk for harm from exposure to RF energy because RF energy can reach a larger area of a child's brain than that of an adult's.

A child's brain and body grow and develop through the teen years. During this time, the body may be more easily affected by RF energy and the effect may be more harmful and longer lasting.

A child who uses a cell phone will have many more years of exposure to RF energy in his or her lifetime than someone who started using a cell phone as an adult.

There is not a lot of research about the effects of cell phone RF energy on children or teenagers, but a few studies have shown that there may be hearing loss or ringing in the ears, headaches, and decreased general well-being.

continued from page 113

The Truth Is . . .

Don't sleep with your phone . . .

- Better yet, move it to another room, or at least as far away as possible. And, you guessed it, double check that WiFi and Bluetooth are off.

Take off the headset when you're not on a call.

- One correction. Headsets release LARGE amounts of radiation, even when you are not using your phone. I have never measured one that was in the safe range. And my meters indicate that bursts of radiation occur every 6-30 seconds on average.

Don't rely on a "radiation shield" . . .

- This is true. I have tested many shields. People think, falsely, that the shields protect them. But there are always one or more "holes" in the case to let calls come through. And if calls come through, radiation goes out.

What about children?

- Children: The statement makes important points that I agree with. However, the truth is that there are a LOT of studies about the effect of digital devices on young people, and it involves much more than "decreased general well-being."

continued from page 107

Shortly after the release of the California Department of Public Health report, the "pushback" appeared, creating more confusion, or perhaps "comfort"—nothing to worry about after all.

Here is the next day's headline:

California: Here's how to handle unfounded fears of cell phone cancer. There's still no solid evidence that cell phones pose any risk.

The article states that, "The main concern by some public health researchers is that radiofrequency energy from cell phones may cause cancers, particularly brain cancers. Yet, there's no clear mechanism that would justify this concern." (Mole, 2017)

It goes on to detail the difference between ionizing and non-ionizing radiation, claiming that radiation is harmful only when producing heat.

The author says there are a "few" studies that might indicate a connection between EMR and brain cancer, but that the studies couldn't be replicated. I challenge that statement with the research that I have plodded through in preparing to write this book. It is neither "few" nor uncompelling. And I haven't even scratched the surface.

You might want to review, "He Said, She Said" in Chapter 3 for some reasons for conflicting reports. The reader will have to determine what is fiction or fact. And consider the source.

In the telling words of astronomer Carl Sagan:

Absence of evidence is not evidence of absence.

But the industry isn't the only one neglecting or minimizing the truth. While we'd like to blame big business, we as consumers are also to blame. We, as a culture, are obsessed with and attached to our electronic devices as if our lives depend on them. We fear missing a CALL or TEXT more than we fear

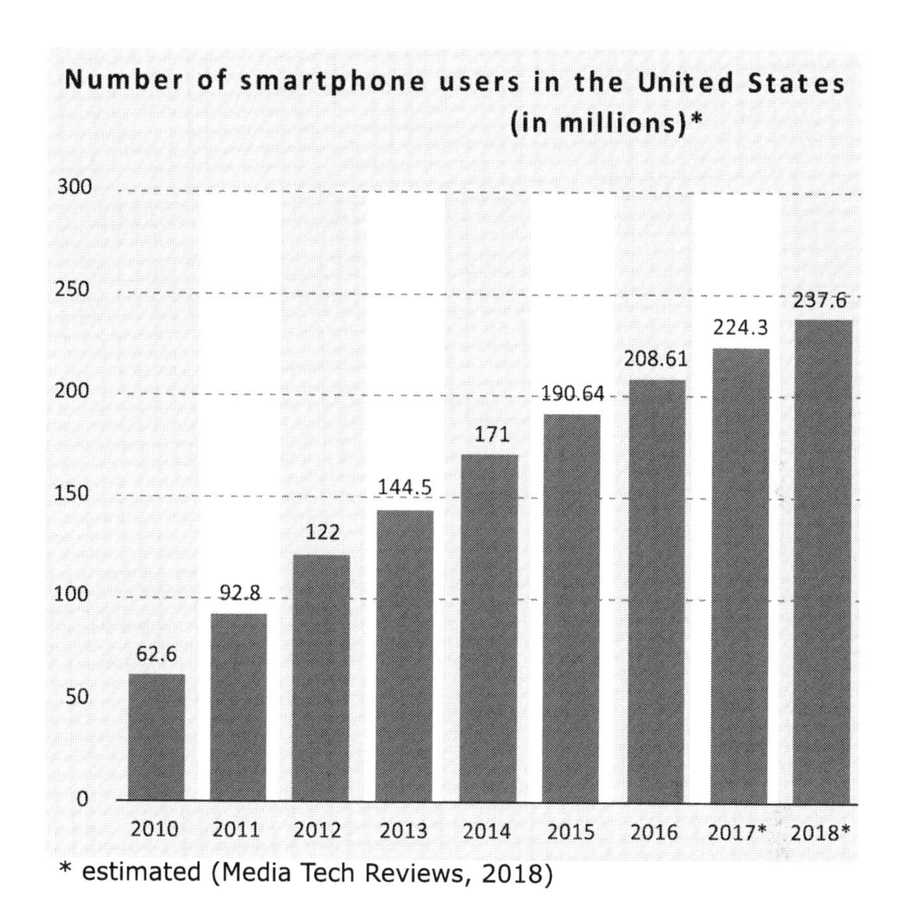

* estimated (Media Tech Reviews, 2018)

missing our birthdays or anniversaries. We are naturally suspicious of information suggesting our favorite things might have deleterious effects on our health.

Technology is not just a personal habit of convenience—it has become necessary in business and connecting with others in our modern way of life. Our dependence on electronics has become deeply ingrained. Even as I prepare this book, I am depending on electronics. And I wouldn't have it any other way.

Fortunately, I am heeding my own advice in Section II—using a wired computer, keyboard, and mouse, and my wired printer is turned OFF, unless in use. The rolling desk upon which my PC sits is pulled away from the wires in the wall. My cell phone is placed across the room. My exposure to all types of hazardous electromagnetic radiation (through the air and from the wires) has been dialed way back.

None of us want to hear bad news about our favorite habits, whether it's food or phones. But there ARE steps we can take to reduce our exposure to harmful EMR/EMF. Some instances may require a little sacrifice and creativity, such as not employing certain devices, or substituting alternative, low-EMF tools for the current trends. However, there are many ways you can use existing technology in a safer way. What is your health, your family's health, and even your pet's health worth? (See Section II: The Solutions Are Doable.)

"It's time to say it out loud," says Larry Gust, BBEC, EMRS. "It's not just the RF from your cell that's a concern—it's everything taken together. It's the RF mesh that's everywhere, created by all these sources. Safe levels of RF, according to studies of health effects, are getting harder to find."

Why isn't everyone sounding the alarm?

Money, Money, Money!

Money buys influence, including at the research level.

The Business Dictionary defines lobbying as: The act of attempting to influence business and government leaders to create legislation or conduct an activity that will help a particular organization.

Who is involved in the Telecommunications Industry?

The Telecommunications Industry: Also known as the "telecom" business, this industry includes all business dealing with the transmission of information, words, sounds, images, or videos, usually over great distances, in the form of electromagnetic signals. It includes wired and wireless industries.

Electronics Manufacturing: Companies that develop and manufacture electronics dealing with electrical circuits that involve active electrical components (such as transistors, diodes,

This is a list, from The Center for Responsive Politics, of lobbying money and its sources, as of 2019:

Industry	Total
Pharmaceuticals/Health Products	$295 million
Electronics Mfg & Equip	$156 million
Oil & Gas	$125 million
Business Associations	$121 million
Electric Utilities	$118 million
Insurance	$117 million
Hospitals/Nursing Homes	$107 million
Misc. Mfg & Distributing	$105 million
Air Transport	$104 million
Securities & Investment	$100 million
Telecom Services	$100 million
Health Professionals	$ 95 million
Health Services/HMOs	$ 89 million
Real Estate	$ 88 million
Education	$ 81 million
Civil Servants/Public Officials	$ 75 million
Internet	$ 74 million
Automotive	$ 69 million
Commercial Banks	$ 61 million
Defense Aerospace	$ 46 million
Telephone Utilities	$ 31 million

(CRP, OpenSecrets.org, 2019)

integrated circuits, optoelectronics, and sensors), associated passive electrical components, and interconnection technologies.

Electric Utilities: An electric utility is a company in the electric power industry that engages in the generation and distribution of electricity. An electric power system is a group of generation, transmission, distribution, communication, and other facilities that are physically connected.

The Internet: The vast computer network linking computer networks worldwide. It is a network of networks that consists of private, public, academic, business, and government networks of local to global scope, linked by a broad array of electronic, wireless, and optical networking technologies.

Telecommunication Services: A telecommunications service is a service provided by a telecommunications provider, also called a "carrier," for a specified set of user-information transfer capabilities provided to a group of users by a telecommunications system.

At first glance, it appears that the pharmaceuticals/health products are the big money wielders at $295 million.

However, if you lump together all the industries associated with telecommunications and electric utilities, it reveals the powerful punch of lobbyists throwing cash at government officials and our elected representatives.

Electronics Mfg & Equip	$156 million
Electric Utilities	$118 million
Telecom Services	$100 million
Internet	$ 74 million
Telephone Utilities	$ 31 million
Total	**$479 million**

(Statistics Portal, retrieved 2019)

And that is just one stream of currency in the U.S. lobbying efforts. I suspect there are a lot more currents of monetary influence.

Just how much money are we talking about? In 2016, the revenue for the telecom industry in the U.S. was close to $256 billion. A year later, in 2017, revenues generated from all sectors of this market had grown to roughly $266 billion. One projection has the U.S. telecom market size reaching $1.3 trillion by 2020. (Radiant Insights, 2016)

The money is globally e-NOR-mous. The global revenue made from telecom services is expected to reach almost 2.4 trillion Euros in 2019 (roughly US$2.88 trillion). The fastest-growing telecommunications services market, with an estimated value of 372 billion Euros in 2016, is the Asia-Pacific region, followed by North America and Europe, according to Insight Research Corporation. (Insight Research, 2014)

The telecommunication services market is made up of two main services: wired and wireless. The largest telecom operators in the world are currently two American multinational corporations: AT&T, headquartered in Dallas, Texas, and Verizon Communications, based in New York. Other strong players include China Mobile (China), Deutsche Telekom (Germany), and Orange (France). (Statistics Portal, retrieved 2018)

Follow the money. When the tobacco industry battled the negative outcry against cigarettes, their goal was to . . . Just create DOUBT. Create doubt about the causation of cancer. And it succeeded for decades.

When the pressure of evidence mounted, the tobacco companies bought more time by affirming that although they believed their products to be safe, just in case, they had added a new filter, made out of asbestos, for worry-free smoking. And of course, they were always happy to fund more research. And so they stalled. All the while, they sucked in huge amounts of money and generated large profits. Profit before people. The government reluctantly edged up a warning or two, that cigarettes "may" be hazardous to one's health.

Similarly, we see the telecommunications industry tossing out a few bones to those who may be concerned . . . just in case. Just in case.

And the government isn't saying much, unless forced to.

Why isn't everyone sounding the alarm?

Some ARE!

Some countries ARE sounding the alarm and passing laws to protect young children. There is growing concern internationally about this ubiquitous, unseen, and largely untested health hazard.

Here are a few examples from around the world. For a more complete update, check out Environmental Health Trust Database of Worldwide Policies on Cell Phones, Wireless and Health: ehtrust.org/policy/international-policy-actions-on-wireless/, and Parents for Safe Technology: norad4u.blogspot.com.

France

2011 French Cell Phone Statute: Requires merchants to display SAR (specific absorption rate) levels for different phone models; all phones must be sold with a headset; bans cell phone ads aimed at children younger than 14.

2013 report on WiFi: The National Agency for Health, Food and Environmental Safety (ANSES) issued a report on the science of the technology.

2015 law passed: WiFi banned from nursery schools; and in elementary schools, WiFi must be turned off when not in use.

A number of libraries, including the French National Library in Paris, and a number of universities and municipal buildings have removed WiFi, or not installed.

A recent headline announced, "France Moves To Ban Students From Using Cellphones In Schools." France's education chief says that when students go back to school in the fall of 2018, all mobile phone use will be banned in schools for students roughly 15 years old and younger. (Wamsley, 2017)

Belgium

Federal public health regulations were issued in 2013 due to health concerns for children. Phones designed for children under seven years old are prohibited from sale. Advertising for cell phones aimed at children younger than 14 is banned.

Warning label on phones: "Think about your health—use your mobile phone moderately . . ."

Recommendations include use of hands-free methods to keep the phone away from the body, such as text messaging, and not making calls when the signal is weak, such as in elevator or vehicle. (Furniere, 2018)

Spain

The Parliament of Navarra voted to urge removal of WiFi in schools and to apply the precautionary principle in relation to exposure limits to electromagnetic fields whose regulatory levels have become "obsolete."

The parliament voted to adopt a resolution recommending that the standards of exposure to EMR be reviewed and new threshold levels be set for preventative, long-term exposure in all indoor areas.

Israel

The Israeli Ministry of Education has issued guidelines limiting WiFi and cell phone use in schools and has banned the use of wireless networks, Preschool through second grade. A hard-wired direct cable connection is required if the teacher has a computer in the class.

In third and fourth grade classes, Internet use is restricted to three hours per week.

The Education Ministry has instructed all schools to perform radiation tests.

The Health Ministry has called for a halt to WiFi installations. It published "Environmental Health in Israel 2014," which states that "Precautions should be strictly enforced with regard to children, who are more sensitive to developing cancer." and that "wireless communication networks in schools be reduced."

Recommendations from the Israeli Health Ministry:

1. Landline telephones.
2. Use of a speaker while talking on a cell phone.
3. Refraining from installing the base of wireless phones in a bedroom, work room, or children's room.

Australia

The Australian Radiation Protection and Nuclear Safety Agency (ARPANA), in 2013, issued a fact sheet titled "How to Reduce Exposure from Mobile Phones and Other Wireless Devices," recommending decreasing the exposure time and increasing the distance from sources of radiation.

ARPANA recommends that parents encourage their children to "limit their exposure."

Australia has a well-organized advocacy group working to reduce wireless exposures on children. In fact, they have many schools that advertise themselves as intentionally being low-tech.

Italy

In 2012, the Italian Supreme Court ruled that a man's brain tumor was caused by his cell phone use, and that the National Institute for Workmen's Compensation must compensate a worker with a head tumor due to cell phone use. (Alleyne, 2012)

In June 2015, the State Parliament of South Tyrol voted to apply the precautionary principle mandating the state government to:

1. To replace existing wireless networks whenever possible with wired networks in schools, preschools, hospitals, nursing homes, and other public facilities.

2. Establish a working group to assess new technologies and clarify which technologies emit less radiation and provide sustainable technology options.

3. To start an education and awareness campaign that informs about possible health risks, especially regarding the unborn, infants, children, and adolescents.

2017 Decree of the Environment Minister recommends reducing exposure to electromagnetic pollution indoors, as much as possible. Additionally, Italy has one of the strictest distracted driving laws in Europe. (Wyland, 2017)

The Parliamentary Assembly of the Council of Europe

In 2011 the Assembly called on European governments to "take all reasonable measures" to reduce exposure to electromagnetic fields, "particularly the exposure to children and young people who seem to be most at risk from head tumors." The resolution calls for member states to:

1. Implement "information campaigns about the risk of biological effects on the environment and human health, especially targeting children and young people of reproductive age."
2. Reconsider the present standards on exposure to electromagnetic fields and apply ALARA (As Low As Reasonably Achievable) principles.
3. Give preference to wired Internet connections and strictly regulate the use of wireless technology by school children on school property.

Switzerland

The Governing Council of Thurgau Canton recommends for schools to use a wired network instead of a wireless network when the structural makeup of a given school building could accommodate it. (2008)

Germany

The German Federal Ministry for Radiation Protection states that wired networks are to be preferred over wireless.

In 2007, parliament recommended not to install wireless networks in schools.

Austria

Gerd Oberfeld, MD, of the Public Health Department of the Salzburg Region, advises not to use WiFi and cordless phones in Schools or Kindergartens."

The Austrian Medical Society issued cell phone safety guidelines stating that cell phones should be used for as short of a time as possible and that children under 16 should not use cell phones at all. In March 2012, the Austrian Medical Association recognized and developed Electromagnetic Hypersensitivity (EHS) diagnosis and treatment guidelines.

United Kingdom

The UK National Health Service issued guidelines and recommendations for children and cell phones, warning that children should only use mobile phones for emergencies and keep all calls short.

The NHS also recommends keeping the phone away from the body and on standby mode, only using it when the reception is strong. "Mobile phone safety – Risks" is featured on the UK National Health Service website.

European Environment Agency (EEA)

Professor Jacqueline McGlade, the EEA's executive director, said, "Recent research and reviews on the long-term effects of radiations from mobile telecommunications suggest that it would be prudent for health authorities to recommend actions to reduce exposures, especially to vulnerable groups, such as children."

The EEA issued a report in 2011 stating that precautionary actions would limit the size and seriousness of any brain tumor risk that may exist.

UE (United Europe)

2011: A Council of Europe committee examined evidence that telecommunications technologies have "potentially harmful" effects on humans, and concluded that immediate action was required to protect children.

In a report, the committee said it was crucial to avoid repeating the mistakes made when public health officials were slow to recognize the dangers of asbestos, tobacco smoking, and lead in petrol (gasoline). (Looks like they took the Walk Down Memory Lane seriously.) The report also highlighted the potential health risks of cordless telephones and baby monitors, which rely on similar technology. (Gray, 2011)

India

2012: the Ministry of Communications and Information Technology issued EMF Guidelines, dropping exposure limits to one tenth of the level suggested by the International Commission on Non-Ionizing Radiation Protection (ICNIRP), and instituted SAR labeling on cell phones.

Official guidelines for cell phone use include: headsets, speakerphones, limiting cell use, increasing distance from devices, and choosing landlines.

2013: Supreme Court of India upheld the High Court of the State of Rajasthan decision to remove all cell towers from the vicinity of schools, hospitals, and playgrounds because of radiation "hazardous to life."

The members of the State Legislature and Parliament of India (Zila Parishad) ordered removal of all cell phone towers near schools, citing exposure to "harmful radiation."

India has some of the strictest exposure limits for EMF radiation in the world.

Russia

The Russian National Committee on Non-Ionizing Radiation Protection has repeatedly warned about electromagnetic radiation impacts on children and recommended WiFi not be used in schools.

In its 2008 report, the committee stated, "The members of the Russian National Committee on Non-Ionizing Radiation Protection emphasize the urgency to defend children's health from the influence of the EMF of the mobile communication systems. We appeal to the government authorities, to the entire society, to pay closest attention to this coming threat and to take adequate measures in order to prevent negative consequences to the future generation's health."

Canada

Health Canada offers "Practical Advice" on reducing exposure to wireless radiation.

2015: National Bill C-648 introduced into the House of Commons: "An Act Respecting the Prevention of Potential Health Risks From Radiofrequency Electromagnetic Radiation." It would require manufacturers of all wireless devices to place specific health warning labels clearly on packaging. As of this writing, there has been no apparent action taken on this bill.

Finland

The Radiation and Nuclear Safety Authority, in 2009, and again in 2015 issued recommendations for reducing children's exposure to EMFs which include:

1. favoring text messages
2. parents limiting duration and amount of calls
3. the use of hands free devices
4. avoiding calls in a low reception area
5. keeping the phone away from the body.

"With children, we have reason to be especially careful, because there is not enough research on children's mobile phone use," stated Dr. Sisko Salomaa, professor of radiobiology at University of Eastern Finland, and former research director of the Radiation and Nuclear Safety Authority in Finland (STUK).

2017: WiFi OFF Switches Installed in the Fiskars primary school.

Cyprus

October 2015: The Cyprus National Committee on Environment and Child Health (ECH) announced it wanted "to err on the side of caution," warning the public that using mobile devices could be potentially harmful to children.

Stella Michaelidou, president of the ECH, warns, "Documentation of other potential and more serious biological side effects are on the tip of an emerging iceberg."

2017 The Minister of Culture and Education directs a ban of WiFi from kindergarten and elementary school classrooms.

The Cyprus National Committee on Environment and Children's Health has produced a brief but powerful video that's worth watching: tinyurl.com/ExposedCyprus. It's in Greek. But there are graphics and subtitles. Looks like this small country has a big concern for its children. "Opa!"

United States

Legislation has been introduced at the state and national levels. Some communities have issued proclamations and resolutions, and started initiatives to inform the public of the health hazards of wireless technology. But only a few actions have actually been passed and implemented, mostly because of the efforts of grassroots health advocates.

2010: San Francisco, California: Cell Phone Radiation (How to Reduce Exposures) website launches. San Francisco develops a poster, factsheet, and display stickers.

2011: The San Francisco Cell Phone Right to Know Ordinance requires cell phone retailers to distribute an educational sheet created by the San Francisco Department of

Environment that explains radio-frequency emissions from cell phones and how consumers can minimize their exposure. The CTIA sued the city to block implementation of the ordinance arguing that the ordinance goes against Federal Communications Commission oversight of standards that keep phones safe. The city settled with the CTIA in exchange for a waiver of attorneys' fees. The city's Cell Phone Radiation webpage remains online. San Francisco developed a poster, factsheet, and display stickers. Wow! Just wow! If you glossed over the above paragraph as I first did, read it again. Look for the money, power, and influence.

2012: Jackson Hole, Wyoming, issues a Proclamation of Cell Phone Safety, which cites concern over long-term health effects as well as the increased risk the radiation poses to children.

2012: Pembroke Pines, Florida, passes Resolution 3362 expressing the city's "Urgent Concerns" about Wireless Radiation and Health. It encourages citizens to read their owner's manuals, and presents information on how to reduce exposure.

2012: Congress, House of Representatives propose legislation: The Cell Phone Right to Know Act, H.R. 6358, is introduced, receiving strong support from many organizations, including the American Academy of Pediatrics. This legislation called for labels on mobile devices at point of sale, a comprehensive national research program to study whether exposure to wireless devices causes adverse biological effects, to be directed by the National Institute of Environmental Health Sciences (NIEHS) and the EPA. It also calls for exposure-level regulation. (The FCC currently has "standards" but no "regulations." I could not find any action taken on this bill.)

2013: Activists in Sedona, Arizona, successfully blocked the blanketing of its community with electric utility smart meters not only by pressuring officials to allow rate payers to opt out of the program, but to refund fees rate payers had paid to opt out.

2014: Wireless Router Labeling in all Suffolk, New York Public buildings. The Suffolk County Legislature passed legislation to require all county buildings to post notices that wireless routers are in use, such as, "Notice: Wireless technology in use."

2014: Greenbelt, Maryland: The city council voted unanimously in November 2014 to alert citizens about the fine-print warnings and possible health risks of cell phones and wireless devices, and to send the FCC chairman a letter urging the adoption of "radiation standards that will protect human health and safety." They also voted to oppose cell towers on school grounds.

2015: Berkeley, California requires cell phone retailers to provide those who purchase a new phone an informational fact sheet that urges buyers to read the user manual to learn the cell phone's minimum separation distance from the body.

2016: School districts begin to adopt best practices for technology. Includes turning off devices when not in use, and placing laptops and tablets on tables.

2017: Maryland State Children's Environmental Health and Protection Advisory Council recommends Wired Internet In Schools.

2017: Under pressure, California Department of Public Health publishes, "How to Reduce Exposure to Radiofrequency Energy from Cell Phones."

2017: A groundswell of grassroots concern delays 5G implementation in California.

Interestingly, most of the concern and movement on the topic of EMF in the United States is from local and grassroots movements, not from government agencies.

Are you wondering why there isn't more legislative action in the U.S.? Especially concerning cell towers near or even on school grounds? According to Section 704 of the 1996 Telecommunications Act, local zoning may be pre-empted by the FCC. Your local community does not have the authority to determine zoning when it comes to wireless infrastructure. Period.

International summary

Mary Redmayne, PhD and Adjunct Research Fellow at Victoria University of Wellington, New Zealand, states that because there is a sufficient body of scientific evidence, "I think it can be agreed upon that the highly complex nature of both RF-EMF and the human body, and frequent technological updates, means simple assurance of long-term safety cannot be guaranteed. . . ."

In the article, published in *Electromagnetic Biology and Medicine* (2015), Redmayne urges that ICNIRP guidelines publish how the head, torso, and limbs' exposure limits were calculated, and what safety margin was applied since this exposure, especially to the abdomen, is now dominant in many children.

Worldwide Precautionary Action

Around the world, countries are taking strong action to reduce wireless radiation on children.

Such countries as Switzerland, Italy, France, Austria, Luxembourg, Bulgaria, Poland, Hungary, Israel, Russia, and China have set RF exposure limits 100 to 10,000 times less than the United States. These countries recognize that there can be non-thermal biological effects from wireless radiation. (Parents For Safe Technology, retrieved 2018)

We SHOULD sound the alarm.

If EMR Is so Dangerous, Why Isn't Everyone Sick?

The argument is often made that IF there is a serious health hazard from the use of cell phones, most everyone would be sick because almost everyone uses cell phones. And, surely, the government would not allow an unsafe product or practice to proliferate our country. Surely.

The research has clearly shown reason for concern. I'm afraid that by the time the cancers and other diseases really explode, it will be too late. The infrastructure for 5G and its related technologies will be deeply imbedded, and our commerce and culture will be largely dependent upon it. Sick will be the new normal. Well, maybe it already IS. Don't confuse longevity charts with wellness.

Recalling the Chernobyl tragedy, the magnitude of that crisis was not that thousands died in one day, but that millions have had their health eroded over time.

Similarly, electro-pollution may not simultaneously slay thousands in a single day. Instead, it slowly erodes our health and makes us all vulnerable to a host of diseases, the onset of which may take years. Maybe that is why it is so easy to overlook this menacing, invisible force.

Give It Another 5-10 Years!

The next generation is at tremendous risk for serious physical diseases and already IS experiencing a host of mental and emotional disorders.

Back to Chapter 3—one analysis projected a tsunami of brain cancer incidence in approximately 15 years. This projection was based on well-established effects of cell phone radiation on DNA mutations, along with the finding that mobile phone use decreases the efficiency of the repair of mutated DNA.

The research paper, by Martin Blank, PhD, and Reba M. Goodman, PhD, and titled "Electromagnetic fields and health: DNA-based dosimetry," was published by *Electromagnetic Biology and Medicine*, June 7, 2012.

Lloyd Morgan, a UC Berkeley researcher and safety advocate, said, "What this analysis shows is that, unless mobile phone usage behavior patterns significantly change, we can reasonably expect a pandemic of brain tumors, for which we are ill-prepared, beginning approximately 15 years from now." And that was in 2012. (Mercola, 2012)

There are reasons I believe it is coming sooner than later:

1. Each generation (G) of phone is more powerful than the previous one.
2. There are more and more cell towers and wireless signals stacking up, layer upon layer in our environment.
3. Usage has increased. How much do you use wireless technology now compared with 5 years ago?
4. Age of users is getting younger, and WiFi is prevalent in schools.

We don't really know how this is going to turn out.

Take note next time you are in a store, or sitting in an office, how many young children have a phone to their heads or have a tablet inches from their faces or abdomens.

Aren't we proud of these technological abilities? Look how "smart" our children are! And see how quietly they sit while they live-stream educational video games.

Yes . . . but . . . a child's brain is so very vulnerable to radiation. A child's DNA is still more easily damaged than an adult's. The immune system is still building and can be tragically impaired. How much control do we have over DDT—Dosage, Distance, Time of exposure?

And that's just the physical harm. Social and psychological digital damage is real and heartbreaking. Recent brain imaging studies conclusively show that excessive screen exposure can neurologically damage a young person's developing brain in the same way that cocaine addiction can. I would suggest that we are already in a serious health crisis in that regard. (Kardaras, 2016; Huddleston, 2016)

How do we know if someone will acquire an illness? Genetic predisposition and individual susceptibility are important factors in the equation.

Think of it like this. We all have been given a gun. It's a revolver. That gun has a cylinder full of bullets representing diseases we could potentially get under the wrong conditions. Think of offending environmental factors as what pulls the trigger. Which bullet will the hammer strike? What constitutes your "wrong conditions" that trigger a genetic predisposition to a particular disease? Could EMR be your trigger? Maybe not. But would you play Russian Roulette with your health?

A massive animal study in Italy tested the effects of low levels of non-ionizing radiation in conjunction with already existing carcinogens. It was determined that EMR enhanced the negative effects of the carcinogens.

The study, carried out at the Ramazzini Institute in Bologna, Italy, concluded that: "The main result of our experiment is that ELF (Extremely Low Frequency) EMFs have a synergistic effect: They are able to enhance the effects of a well-known carcinogen at low doses that was negative at those doses in the same experimental model." (Microwave News, 2016)

It is possible that someone who has a genetic predisposition to a particular disease, and who has also been exposed to carcinogenic agents, may experience enhanced sensitivity to the promotional effects of electromagnetic fields. (Keen, 2015)

What body burdens are present in your life? What elements in your environment could have a potentiating effect on any familial physical weaknesses?

Why isn't everyone sick? Maybe we are and we just don't know it yet. Maybe disease will rear its ugly head later in life. Or perhaps our genetic makeup is strong enough to defend us from disease.

EHS—Electromagnetic Hypersensitivity

My wife is so sensitive to fragrances and chemicals that when she walks down the detergent aisle of the grocery store, she feels pain and pressure behind her eyes.

My sensitivity is to smoke. I can be sick for many days after having been in the vicinity of a forest fire. And diesel exhaust can wreak havoc on my sinuses.

Maybe you have certain allergies or sensitivities that trigger symptoms such as sneezing or a headache or nausea.

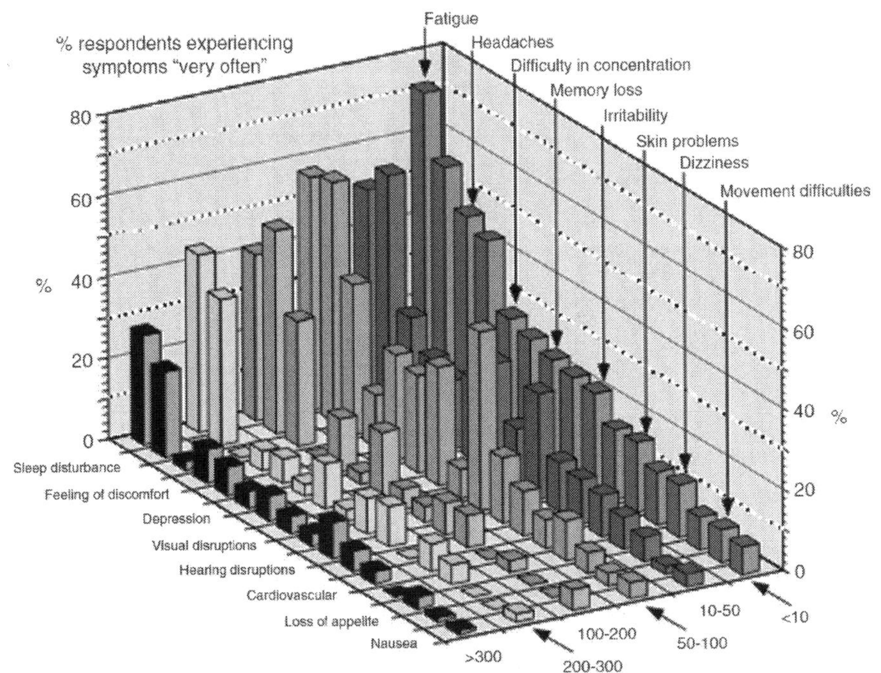

Symptoms experienced by people near cellular phone base stations. (Havas, 2013) [Based on the work of Santini et al., 2003. Reprinted with permission of Magda Havas.]

Imagine being surrounded by the offensive trigger day and night, wherever you go.

EMR sensitivity is a difficult malady. There are people so sensitive that when they walk into a home, they can immediately tell if you have your cell phone on or off. They can feel it if your router is on. They cannot walk into a big box store without feeling dizzy and sick. And some even hear sounds associated with electricity, such as "buzzing," or "high-pitched humming."

People who suffer from Electromagnetic Hypersensitivity (EHS) experience symptoms when exposed to non-ionizing electromagnetic radiation. Symptoms vary widely, and the most commonly reported include headaches, heart palpitations, pressure in the chest, extreme fatigue, stress, tinnitus (ringing in the ears), skin symptoms ranging from rashes to burning sensations, pain, muscle aches, issues with memory and concentration, irritability, and sleep disturbances. (Adey, 1993; Blackman, 2007; Belyaev, 2012)

Are you EMF Sensitive? Here are some things to consider:

- Why am I so tired? No, not just tired. Profoundly exhausted. Sigh.
- Do I live with a malaise of undiagnosed, vague symptoms?
- Why am I worse in certain rooms or locations?
- Is there a place where my symptoms are particularly worse?
- Do I feel better when I am away from my home?
- Is there a place where my symptoms recede or disappear altogether?
- Do my symptoms go away when I am visiting other geographical locations?

In her book *Zapped* (2010), Ann Louise Gittleman makes a compelling case for EMR causing "subliminal, or stealth stress." This stress has been shown to interrupt communication between the body's cells and can result in a host of unintended consequences for the EHS person. Remember, man-made EMR is not found in nature and is, therefore, "foreign" to the human body. Some seem to handle it OK, or at least we think we do. But others are desperately ill. It is as if an EHS person is "allergic" to non-ionized EMR.

With the permeation of wired and wireless infrastructure, it becomes increasingly difficult to escape second-hand EMF exposure. If you are sitting on a subway or waiting for a concert or sporting event to start, how many people in your periphery have some sort of electronic device invisibly polluting your space? As for work spaces, how many people have the flexibility to move their desks to a wall that has minimal radiation emanating from the wiring hidden inside the walls, if such a place can even be found? Then there is the proliferation of office equipment and WiFi in most business environments. It becomes very tricky, if not impossible, for an EMR-sensitive person to find a suitable work environment. That holds true for many social environments, as well.

One of the world's leading experts on EHS (electromagnetic hypersensitivity) is Lloyd Burrell. He has lived through the malaise of this potentially debilitating response to EMFs. In his own quest for wellness, Lloyd has interviewed hundreds of health professionals to come up with practical solutions to cope with environmental challenges and to promote healing. His book, *EMF Practical Guide: The Simple Science of Protecting Yourself, Healing Chronic Inflammation, and Living a Naturally Healthy Life in Our Toxic Electromagnetic World* (2019), is an outstanding resource for anyone, but particularly for those who are suffering from EHS

At the 2009 Southwest Conference on Disability in Albuquerque, New Mexico, Pamela Reed Gibson discussed this conundrum of EHS from a social-emotional-psychological perspective, identifying the resultant isolation that often follows. Her article, "The Hidden Marginalization of Persons with Environmental Sensitivities," was published in *Ecopsychology* in 2016.

With 5G now a reality, it will be almost impossible to escape the tidal wave of electro-pollution. The challenge is great.

In 2015, a group of nearly 200 scientists representing 40 countries presented a written appeal to the United Nations and World Health Organization to give more attention to the dangers of EMR. Among their recommendations was recognizing and educating health professionals about people with EHS and the creation of EMR "safe zones."

There are a few communities in the United States that are described as EMF Quiet Zones:

United States National Radio Quiet Zone—Green Bank, West Virginia.

Originally created by the Federal Communications Commission (FCC) in 1958 to protect the radio telescopes in Green Bank and Sugar Grove, the United States National Radio Quiet Zone has become a safe haven for many who suffer from electromagnetic hypersensitivity. It includes 13,000 square miles that spans West Virginia, Virginia, and a small part of Maryland. Due to the sensitivity of the telescopes, wireless technology is banned within the zone, and radio, cellular, and other broadcast transmissions are restricted to certain frequencies.

The few allowed transmitters operate at reduced power using highly directional antennas. This makes it an ideal refuge for many severe EHS sufferers who find themselves able to live more of a normal life inside the Quiet Zone.

Snowflake MCS/EHS Community—Snowflake, Arizona

This community comprises a few dozen people suffering from severe MCS (multiple chemical sensitivities) and electrical sensitivities and who live in close proximity. The area is mostly rural and mostly zoned for 20 acres per house, so there is little electro-pollution from neighbors. The levels of electro-pollution in Snowflake are generally low; there is one cell tower in Snowflake, with the next closest tower a few miles away.

The Quiet Dome—Grass Valley, California

Built to be electromagnetically quiet, the dome is situated far from cell towers or WiFi in the Sierra Nevada Mountains. "The dome has no WiFi (it has wired Internet), no cell towers within two miles, clean power (harmonics are filtered out), and silent appliances (all lighting is direct current)." The dome was built by someone who developed many environmental and food sensitivities at age 15 after having dental work for a gold bridge placed next to existing mercury fillings. In addition to being electrosmog-free, the dome is built with non-toxic and mold-hostile materials, and intended to provide a place for EHS sufferers to detox and recover.

ElectroMagnetic Sensitivity Research Institute—Rockvale, Colorado

The ElectroMagnetic Sensitivity Research Institute (EMSRI) is working on the development of safe housing for those with sensitivities. The initiative was started by Dr. Gary Johnson, who purchased 59 acres in Rockvale, Colorado, which includes a gulch shielded from electromagnetic waves on three sides by topography. The EMSRI is currently actively looking for people to help with the initiative, including researchers, medical people, people suffering from EMF sensitivities, and investors.

Wisconsin

Lynn Knapp purchased low-EMF acreage in southwest Wisconsin and wants to create an electro-safe community for other EMF refugees. Knapp says, "I have dealt with EMF for ten years and finally purchased twenty-two acres in southwest Wisconsin that is a safe zone. Feels wonderful there! Looking to create a small community with like folks that are dealing with EMF." (Goldberg, 2015)

Research and awareness is growing. There is plenty of evidence that biological markers can be found for EMF hypersensitivity. (Plourde & Plourde, 2016)

The Austrian Medical Association developed a guideline in 2012 for the diagnosis and treatment of EMF-related health problems and illnesses (EMF syndrome). It includes suggestions for biological testing as well as symptomatic evaluation and a flow chart to track progress in diagnosis and remediation.

However, few health professionals are knowledgeable and sympathetic on treating this disease. And the diagnostic protocol is not well established. Yet.

If you are ill, and have no discernible cause, it seems to be a good idea to at least reduce your exposure to disease-causing EMF. Get that off the table.

What's in Your Mouth?

If you believe that you are EHS, it may be a good idea to also address the issue of dental amalgams (silver fillings). Although the American Dental Association and the U.S. government would disagree, there is considerable evidence that heavy metals in your mouth (mercury, nickel, etc.) may affect your sensitivity to EMFs. And that's in addition to the issue of mercury toxicity, which is a whole other topic. (Eggleston, 1984; Paknahad et al., 2016; Mercola, 2017; Deen, 2017)

If you are EHS, you may want to get a heavy-metal test.

Actions for Today:

- ✓ Open your mind to the possibility of EMR/EMF as a serious body burden contributing to EHS and other diseases, and check Appendices II and III for valuable resources.
- ✓ Check out Appendix III for grassroots movements and consider joining.
- ✓ Warn everyone you know about the dangers of constant exposure to radiation from electronics.
- ✓ Be sensitive and thoughtful to those in your vicinity who may be EHS.

Need or want solutions right now?

Go to Chapters 7, 8 and 9 (more than 30 pages of solutions) and Appendix I for your Comprehensive Home Safety Audit.

Chapter 6

The Bridge – Time to Cross It

What's your favorite bridge? Mine is Deception Pass Bridge in the San Juan Islands in Washington State. It connects Whidbey Island, where my wife grew up, to Fidalgo Island, which connects to the mainland. I never get tired of crossing over that bridge and taking in the majestic views of Puget Sound on the west side, and the view of snow-capped Mount Baker to the northeast.

I want to encourage you to cross the bridge. Leave the complexity of the EMR/EMF problems and cross over to doing something about them. Section II is all about solutions. It connects you with scientific, measurable solutions. They are doable. And I think you will be pleased at the ease of many of the remedies.

Don't put this off. Start today. Let me add to your sense of urgency.

Picture Barbara. She is in a cold, sterile, doctor's office with her 16-year-old daughter. Katy had been charging her cell phone on her night stand since she was 12 years old. She talked for hours and hours with her teenage friends. She routinely pressed the phone to her ear. And, like most teenagers, she often slept with her phone under her pillow. Now she has a tumor on her face, right where she used to sleep with her cell phone. Sigh . . .

This is a real person living 12 miles from me in Las Vegas, Nevada. Can I prove causation? No. But I wouldn't want to be in that position knowing there were some pretty easy preventative solutions that I could have employed.

Back to Barbara and Katy. The tumor was frightening for both. Thankfully, it was surgically removed, after nine hours of surgery. But a year later the tumor returned and Katy, at age 17, had to have it removed, as well as undergo cosmetic surgery, for another nine hours.

Let's not wait for the government, and media to announce their final verdict on this. Let's not depend on them to guide our course in disease prevention. Remember, it took decades for other hazardous elements to be revealed.

When Rachel Carson took on the chemical industry in her ground-shaking book, *Silent Spring* (1962), she observed that industry leaders possessed "no humility before the vast forces with which they tampered."

In *An Electronic Silent Spring* (2014), author Katie Singer asks some disturbing and relevant questions: "Does our species' survival depend on humbling ourselves? Could we admit how much we do not understand? Could we each acknowledge our electronic footprints?"

We live in a complex world. I think about the intricacies of the human body as I look up at the sign above my computer which reminds me that I am, "fearfully and wonderfully made." (King David, Psalm 139:14; 1,000 BC) And I am humbly reminded how much we do not know.

Admittedly, there are many more questions than answers on this topic of man-made, non-ionizing radiation. And it's true that we don't know what we don't know. But there are some things we can know for sure. One of those things is that there is no evidence proving that the EMR-producing devices that have permeated our space are safe for long-term usage—the way we are currently using them. And there *is* a lot of evidence that they are *not* safe.

Before I knew better, I used to press my cell phone against my ear all of the time. I used to sleep next to a cordless phone base. I also used to eat hot dogs and drink sodas. Used to.

Before my wife knew better, she used to ride her bike for hours with her cell phone turned on in the back pocket of her jersey, directly over her right kidney. She still rides her bike and still carries her phone for emergencies. But with Airplane mode on, and WiFi and Bluetooth off.

We both used to have a mouth full of mercury fillings. Used to. We just didn't know.

Will we get cancer? It's indeterminable. Four of my relatives have died of cancer. Heart disease runs in my wife's family, not cancer. But that's not a sure thing. We've insulted our health so much that anything could happen. And we wouldn't necessarily know which one of the offences was the trigger.

Maybe tomorrow there will be a new study that brings everything into clearer focus. But tomorrow isn't a sure thing any more than our health is.

In the meantime, I choose to apply the Precautionary Principle: Because I know that electromagnetic radiation is harmful to my health, I will take precautionary measures to keep myself, friends and family, and pets as safe as I can, even if some of the cause-and-effect mechanisms are not yet fully understood.

Onward! The next section—How to Protect Yourself—is the most important part of this book. And I'm excited that you are here, about to engage in the solutions.

You might be wondering if I'm going to ask you to give up your electronic devices. In most cases, no. Section II is about using electronics in a safer way.

Maybe you feel that this will take too much time. You are just way too busy. Then you can start with the one-minute solutions, and tackle the more advanced issues later. Like a bicycle seat, small adjustments (up or down, forward or backwards, slight angle of the tilt) can make enormous differences in comfort.

Similarly, small adjustments in the way you use your electronics can make great gains in reducing your exposure to EMR/EMF. People are often amazed when I demonstrate with my meters, how just placing their cell phone across the room dramatically cuts their cell phone radiation exposure. Or, how repositioning their favorite chair away from an electrically "hot" wall brings the radiation numbers way down and into the safe range.

Getting started is as easy as:

✓ Relocating some of your electronics.
✓ Changing what's on your nightstand.
✓ Adopting some new habits.
✓ And possibly a small amount of money.

So, turn the page, and let's get started.

Need or want solutions right now?

Go to Chapters 7, 8 and 9 (more than 30 pages of solutions) and Appendix I for your Comprehensive Home Safety Audit.

SECTION II

How to Protect Yourself—
The Solutions Are Doable

First Steps to an EMF Make-over

Chapter 7

Radiation from WIRES: Fixes Anyone Can Do

Just Say OFF!

Solutions to Electric and Magnetic Radiation are normally the same.

In a nutshell: Unplug or turn OFF whenever possible.

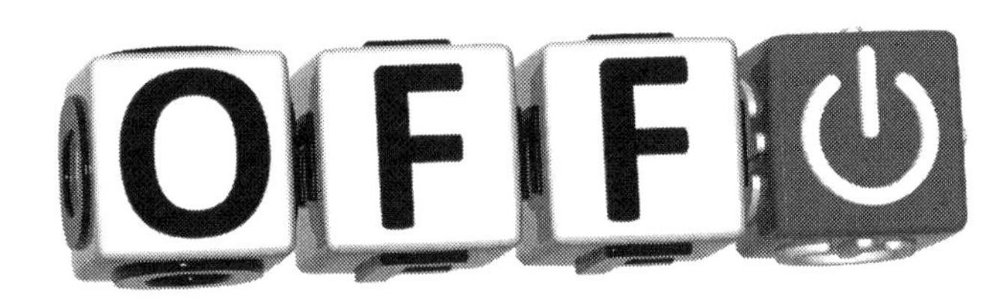

If a device has wireless, WiFi, and/or Bluetooth capability, put it on a power strip and turn off the power strip (cut the power) when not in use. Some devices with wireless, WiFi and/or Bluetooth capability still are producing radiation when they are plugged in, even if you turn the device off.

Don't forget about personal surveillance—the devices can listen, locate, and log your personal and family information. Most smart devices are now designed to collect information when they are plugged in—some even if they are turned off. For more information on this, see **They've Got Us Covered** in Chapter 1.

Unplug or Turn OFF

Don't want to do that?

1. Buy a toggle switch from a hardware store that plugs into the outlet. That will cut off both electric and magnetic

radiation on your favorite lamp under which you sit. Normally, it is the electric field that is the issue with cords. However, wiring errors can cause elevated magnetic fields as well. Unplug any electric cords around your bed or where you sit or stand for extended periods.

2. Even better, you can use a remote-control switch to turn power OFF at the outlet on the wall where you sleep, sit or stand. If you need more plugs, buy a power strip and plug it into the remote control shutoff switch. Make sure you buy the one with three prongs so the power strip can plug into a remote-control shutoff switch. Great for lamps around the bed. Cost? Under $9.00 at a big-box hardware store.
3. You can buy a shielded power strip. Normal power strips generate high Electric Radiation. Consult a Certified Electromagnetic Radiation Specialist on availability since this is a special-order item.

Remember to pull the plug on any kitchen appliances not being used.

Example: I recently did an EMR/EMF home evaluation in a 7,200-square-foot home. The occupants had a home theater with six power recliners. They now have a remote-control power switch to turn off power to the recliners when they are sitting in them. They have dropped their radiation exposure in those power recliners by more than 95 percent. Cost? Under $9.00. Showtime!

This solution is also great for an electric bed. Once it is set up for the night, the power can be turned off with a click of the finger.

Advanced solutions are to have a qualified, EMF-aware electrician replace your two-prong lamp cords with three-prong, shielded cords. Also Low EMR electrical cords are available for purchase. But they need to be installed by an electrician. These things are more expensive, and they require a grounded outlet.

Toggle switches, power cords, remote control outlets, and just pulling the plug are easy and inexpensive solutions to both electric and magnetic radiation.

Distance Is Your Friend

Increase distance from the source. Pull your favorite easy chair away from the wall or electrical cords. Distance is your friend! Remove all electronics from your nightstand and move them across the room.

Example: Our computer is on a rolling desk so that if we are planning on spending a long period of time at the keyboard, we can easily roll it away from the wall where the hidden radiation is emanating from the wires in the wall. And our printer is on a small cart with casters, so it, too, can be pushed away from us when in use. If I'm going to do a quick check of my email, or do a quick search, I leave the setup against the wall. But if I'm planning on spending some time, I roll it out. Works well.

Example: A gourmet candy-making business asked me to come to the business site and do an EMF inspection. I found Lisa standing in a work space that was off the charts in magnetic radiation. By measuring with the right kind of meters, I moved her work area two feet to the right, which dropped her exposure to almost nothing. And the candy is still just as amazing!

Electric and Magnetic Radiation can be measured to ensure safety. This is particularly important for sleeping areas or places where a large amount of time is spent. You may choose to reposition your bed based on Electric and Magnetic Field readings. It's not that hard to do.

Example: Wendy is a young mother concerned about her son's sleeping environment. I mailed her a meter and set up a phone conference appointment; I was able to walk her through the process of metering her child's bedroom. There was one wall that was especially high in magnetic radiation, probably due to it having a wall that had a lot of outlets and wiring. Based on the information she got from measuring, she moved her son's bed to a different wall.

The "offending wall" was still there. But at least her baby's head was not resting on it night after night. Instead of racking up more "zaps," her toddler is safely counting sheep.

And don't forget where your pets are sleeping. Especially if they are near any device has a wireless, WiFi, and/or Bluetooth capability, you will need to put devices on a power strip and turn off the power strip (cut the power) when not in use. Some devices with wireless, WiFi and/or Bluetooth capability still are producing radiation even if you turn the device off.

There are good, better, and best positions for avoiding EMF from the wiring contained in every wall in your home. The best place for a pet bed is away from walls and electrical cords. Remember, 6-8 feet away is the best. But any distance helps. For additional solutions, see Chapter 9.

One measuring device I recommend is the Gigahertz ME3030B. It measures BOTH Electric and Magnetic Radiation by simply flipping a switch and it is easy to use. (See Chapter 10 for more details on meters and Section III, Chapter 12, for charts of "Concern" levels.)

Replace

Get rid of your CFLs (compact fluorescent light bulbs) These include fluorescent tubes and curlicue light bulbs. Dispose of them carefully, according to the EPA hazardous waste recommendations. The EPA recommends that consumers take advantage of available local options for recycling CFLs, fluorescent bulbs, and other bulbs that contain mercury, and all other household hazardous wastes, rather than disposing of them in regular household trash. Large hardware stores (in some states) will handle hazardous disposal for you. Earth 911 has a website where you can find recycling sites near you: earth911.com.

Also, remove LED light bulbs. The blue light emitted from LEDs has been shown to suppress melatonin. They also can produce dirty electricity. I used to think they were OK. I have changed my mind on LEDs. They also flicker like CFLs—the light is not constant. (Bradford, 2016)

Go back to the old-fashioned incandescent light bulbs. If they were good enough for Thomas Edison, they're good enough

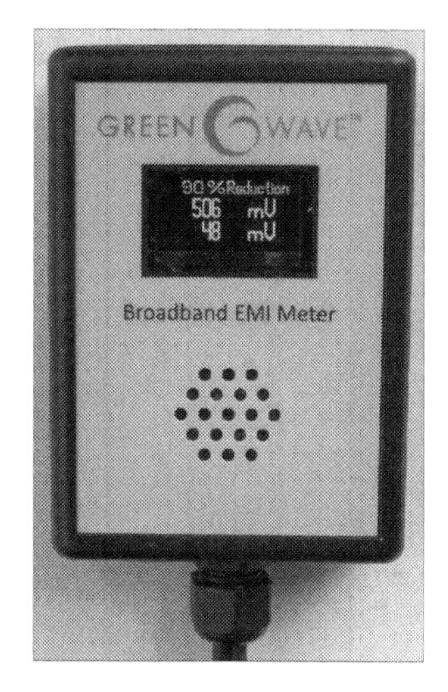

Greenwave meter

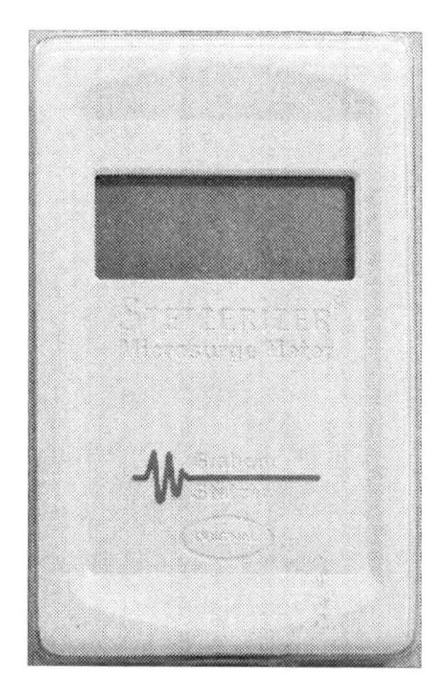

Stetzer meter

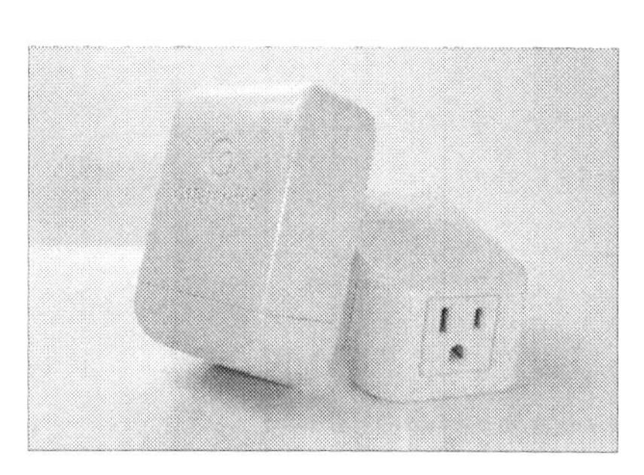

Greenwave filter

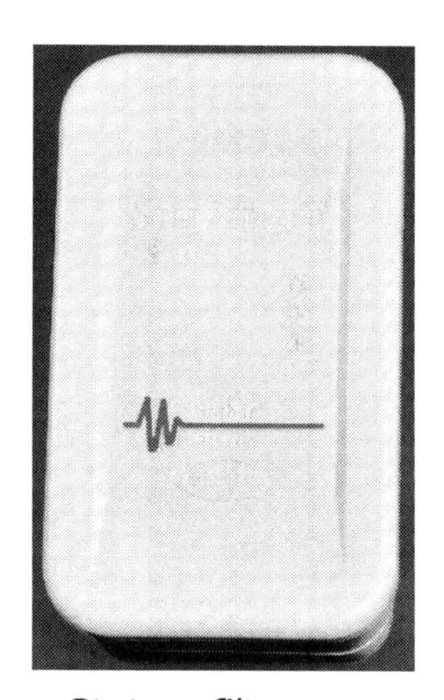

Stetzer filter

for us. These are usually available in lower watt options. For a higher watt option, try Halogen incandescent. Just make sure the bulb has the wide, screw-in base, and not the narrow push-in base.

No dimmers, no dimmers, no dimmers. If you must cling to your mood lights, make sure you turn the switch completely

OFF (not just down) when you are done with your mood. If you are extremely electric-sensitive, you may need to totally remove all dimmers.

Plug It IN

Wait—I thought the idea was to UNplug things. Not in this case.

Dirty electricity (in the technical sense of high-frequency voltage transients and harmonics) is the only type of EMR that can be remediated by plug-in filters or whole-house filters. Whole-house filters are more expensive than the following plug-in filters, so I normally use the plug-in filters.

Solutions to dirty electricity:

✓ Unplug or Turn OFF electronics whenever possible.
✓ Turn Dimmers OFF/No CFL or LED light bulbs.
✓ Increase Distance from sources to 6 to 9 feet.
✓ Plug-in Filters can lower radiation.
✓ Use a Greenwave meter or Stetzer meter to measure. (See Chapter 11 for meter information and Chapter 12 for "Concern" levels.)

In case you missed it, dirty electricity is the only type of EMF that can be remediated by the use of filters. The filters actually deal with the High-Frequency Voltage Transients and Harmonics, or Dirty Electricity (DE), if you prefer.

The filters plug in to your electrical outlets.

There are two different types of filters that I use. There are even ones that provide you with a plug at the bottom so that you don't lose an outlet. Greenwave Filters and Stetzer Filters are both effective in lowering dirty electricity.

They are portable, so we take them with us when we travel to a hotel. And they last a lifetime. We've never found one that lost its effectiveness yet.

Dirty Electricity Advanced Techniques

Sometimes dirty electricity is harder to reduce—especially with solar panels, newer swimming pool pumps with variable speed motors, and also air conditioning and heating systems with variable speed motors.

If you find yourself in this situation you can:

- ✓ Check to see which outlet has the highest dirty electricity in your home.
- ✓ Start with that outlet.
- ✓ If the dirty electricity does not reduce to a reasonable level by just plugging filters into the wall outlets directly, then try a $4 power strip and plug the filters into the power strip. (Levels listed in Chapter 12.)
- ✓ Remeasure the outlets in that room and reduce the next highest outlet in the room with the same techniques.
- ✓ Do these techniques throughout your home

Three Bits of Caution:

1. Dirty electricity filters effectively lower dirty electricity. But on occasion they can raise magnetic fields. You have to check and double check. If this happens, consult a Certified Electromagnetic Radiation Specialist for remediation.
2. There are some electromagnetic hypersensitive people who react better with one filter or the other. If you are EHS, you may want to compare how you feel with both filters and determine which one works best for you. Test them out. If you have a negative reaction, pull them out and try the other type of filter. If neither is right for you, there are other filter options for some EHS people, but they are more expensive. Greenwave has a different type of filter that some EHS people seem to do better with, at the same price.

3. It rarely happens, but if you do feel worse when you plug in dirty electricity filters, remove them and call either a Certified Electromagnetic Radiation Specialist or the manufacturer of the filter for remediation.

Actions for Today:

✓ Take small steps today to reduce the from-the-wires radiation in your home.

✓ Consider using dirty electricity plug-in filters in your sleeping area, office, or work space, and any other area where you spend a lot of time. (It's best to measure and consult with a Certified Electromagnetic Radiation Specialist on this.) To save 5% on Greenwave filters or meters use this code: safe7.

Need or want more solutions right now?

Go to Chapters 8 and 9 and Appendix I for your Comprehensive Home Safety Audit.

Chapter 8

Radiation Through the Air Solutions to Wireless Radiation

First Steps: Ten Ways to Lower Your Exposure to Harmful Radiation

No, not this way!

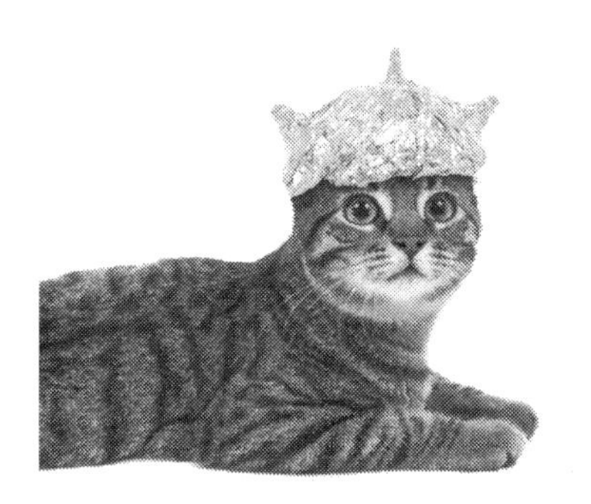

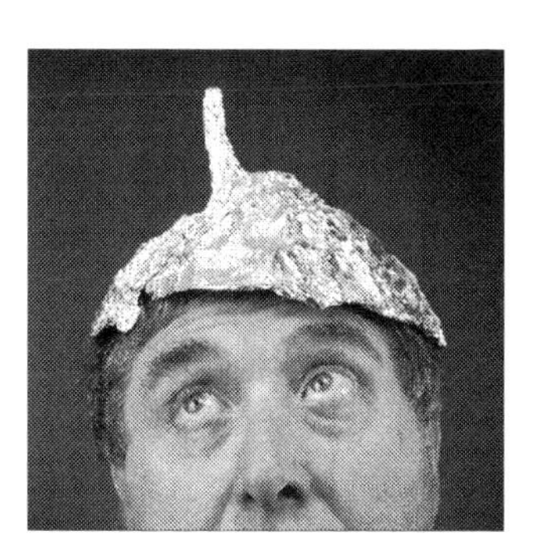

We have scientific, measurable ways to lower your exposure. And the solutions do not annoy pets or make you look weird.

1. Step aWAY from the Microwave!

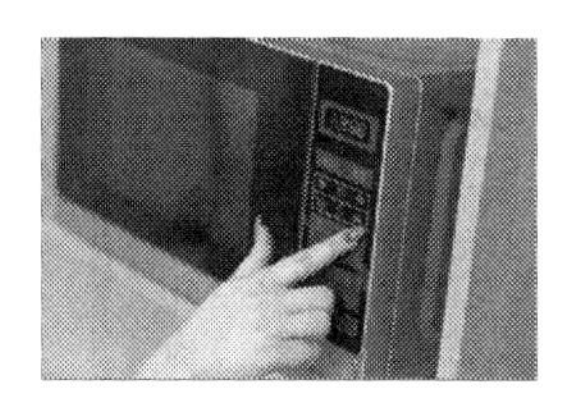

- Microwave ovens generate Wireless Radiation when in use.
- We have never measured a microwave oven that was safe to stand in front of. Why do we do that anyway?
- After starting a microwave oven, get as far away from it as possible.

- ➢ How far is safe? Leave the room and get as far away as possible. And don't forget your pets.

NOTE: Russian studies after WWII demonstrated that microwaving foods had a diminishing effect on the nutritional value.

View the one-minute video "Step Away from the Microwave: Microwave Oven Radiation–How Far to Be Safe?": tinyurl.com/ExposedMicrowave.

Example: I was talking with a retired nurse whose husband had the habit of standing right in front of the microwave when it was in use. I said, "Now you can tell him not to do that." Sadly, she replied, "Too late. He has a huge abdominal tumor." I'm not making any diagnostic claims. But isn't it "better to be safe than sorry"?

2. Move It!

- ✓ Move your cell phone as far away as possible from your sleeping area when charging.
- ✓ Devices that are ON generate Wireless/WiFi/Bluetooth Radiation—even when not being used. Ping-ping-ping. In my measurements, I have observed, on the average, a cell phone tries to connect to the nearest cell tower, WiFi, or Bluetooth device, every six to thirty seconds, even when not making a call. The attempted connections can be hundreds of times the "No Concern" radiation levels. Chargers can generate all types of radiation from the wires. (Electric Radiation, Magnetic Radiation, and Dirty Electricity).
- ✓ Move everything, even clocks and extension cords, away from the nightstand and as far away as possible. (Battery-operated clocks are OK.)

View the one-minute video: "Cell Phone Radiation Danger: Cancer on Your Nightstand; Move Your Cell Phone" tinyurl.com/ExposedNightstand.

Story: Kidney Cancer and Dementia

Meet Betty and Harold. I was at a conference and Betty walked up and told me her husband, Harold, had kidney cancer. I asked her where he carried his cell phone. She said he had clipped his cell phone to his belt, directly over his right kidney. He carried it there for many years, pretty much all day, every day. And that's where he got the cancer.

I can neither prove causation nor promise that he wouldn't have gotten kidney cancer if he had not carried his cell phone there. Still, would you like to be in their shoes, knowing that there were better habits that might have prevented this disaster?

Betty said that since Harold found out he had kidney cancer, he no longer carries it there.

But now Harold has another problem. He's starting to get dementia.

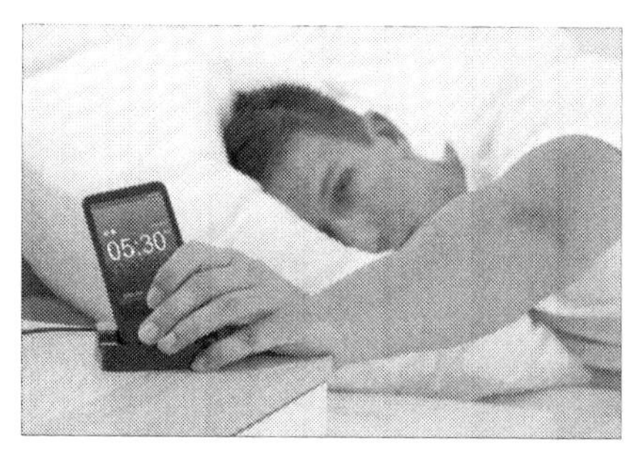

I asked her where he charged his cell phone. Pause. Right on his nightstand, next to his head. Cell phones generate radiation constantly, every 6-30 seconds on the average, even if you are not actively using them. Additionally, the charging cords themselves can produce electric and magnetic radiation as well as dirty electricity. So, he was getting a high dose of all four types of radiation.

Can I say for sure that charging his cell phone on his nightstand was causing his dementia? No. But neither can anyone prove that this is a safe practice.

Move it!

3. Speak Up!

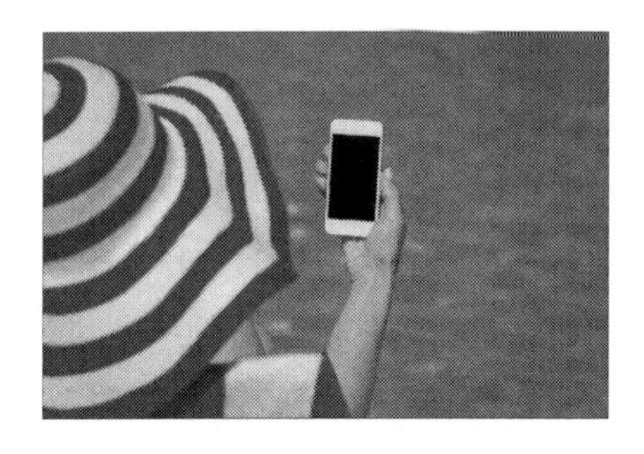

- ✓ Whenever possible, use a cell phone in Speaker mode.
- ✓ Try never to hold a cell phone to your ear.
- ✓ Limit time spent on a cell phone by using a landline when possible.
- ✓ Even industry fine print recommends that a phone should not be pressed against the head.

View the four-minute video: "Cell Phone Radiation Safety Tips With Dr Sanjay Gupta on Anderson Cooper 360": youtube.com/watch?v=v7wCeuSqm34.

4. Up, Up and Away!

When carrying a cell phone on your body or in your purse:

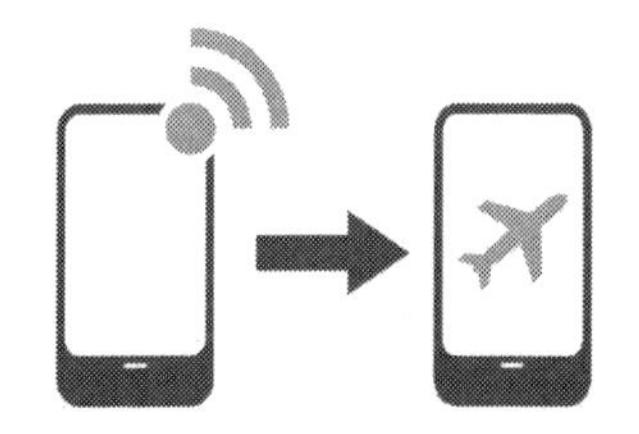

- ✓ Turn Airplane Mode ON.
- ✓ Turn Bluetooth and WiFi OFF.
- ✓ Cell phones generate Radiation even when you are NOT making a call.
- ✓ And don't think that just because the screen is "asleep" that it is not producing radiation.

You must get into the habit of following the above instructions re-li-gious-ly.

Note: In these modes, you will not be able to receive Text, Emails, Data, or Phone calls.

How is this practical? Unless you are expecting an emergency call, it is easy to get in the habit of checking for messages every hour, or more frequently, if you must. Then turn off all the radiation on your phone to safely carry. Admittedly, if you are running a business, you may need to check messages more often. But this will cut down on your exposure to radiation.

Of course, use a landline whenever possible. Then you can place your cell phone as far away as possible.

Why not just turn the phone completely off? You can do that. But then you will not be able to use your camera, calendar, and calculator. Also, it takes less time and less battery power to simply turn on and off Airplane Mode as opposed to powering on and off. Airplane ON, WiFi and Bluetooth OFF. Takes about five seconds.

When you are in the car, place the cell phone on the passenger seat, as far away as possible, assuming you are not in your car for most of the day. If you spend a lot of time in your car, keep phone on airplane mode as much as possible. (And turn WiFi and Bluetooth off.) You can check your messages periodically.

When you get home, place it away from your body—across the room.

Distance is your friend. Small adjustments make great gains in reducing your exposure to radiation.

Another option is to use call forwarding from your cell phone to your landline, if you are home. (Just remember to turn off that feature when you are away from your landline.)

Story: 19-year-old's Hip Replacement

I participated in a continuing education seminar with some of my colleagues in Southern California. The host whose home we were measuring for EMR/EMF said his 19-year-old son had undergone a Total Hip Replacement.

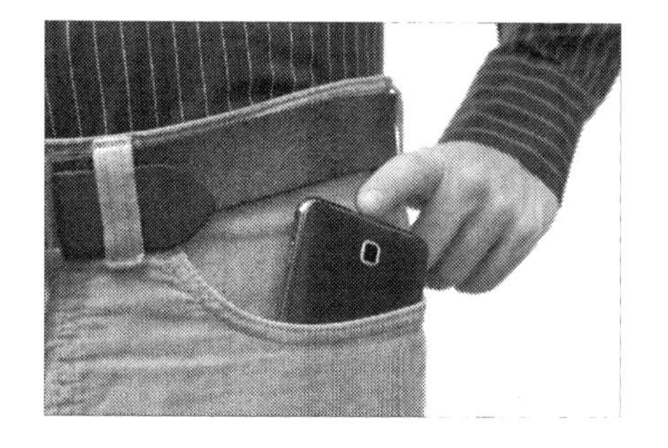

How is it that a 19-year-old young man needed a THR?

Turns out, he started carrying his cell phone in his

front pocket when he was a freshman in high school. All day long that phone stayed tucked away in the same pocket.

When he was 19, he was hiking and jumped off a small rock. His hip shattered. He was rushed to emergency where the surgeon opened him up. The first thing she found was a huge tumor, right where he had carried his cell phone. Once she got through the tumor, she couldn't believe her eyes—she could push her finger right through the bone.

We can't prove that EMR caused the tumor, but it is interesting that the tumor was on same side as where he carried his phone. Would you take that chance? I wouldn't.

I repeat, when carrying a cell phone next to your body:

✓ Turn Airplane Mode ON.

✓ Turn Bluetooth and WiFi OFF.

Some phones automatically shut down WiFi and Bluetooth when placed in airplane mode. Others must be turned off each time. You must check to make sure this is accomplished when carrying your phone next to your body. And this should be checked periodically, as I have found some phones automatically turn these features back on.

5. Rout It Out!

Wireless Router/WiFi/Bluetooth:

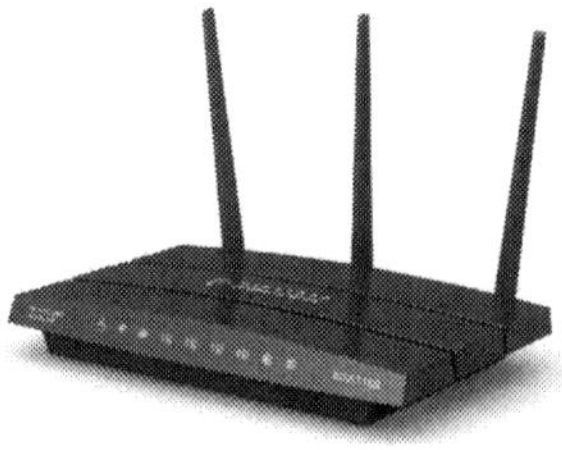

- Generate radiation even when no one is using a portable electronic device.
- Move the router as far away as possible from the living and sleeping areas. Remember, if you have a multi-floor dwelling, the radiation can come right through the floor below you or the ceiling above you.
- The body is trying to rebuild itself when sleeping. WiFi/Wireless/Bluetooth interfere with the process by

suppressing melatonin production. Melatonin suppresses cancer and allows you to get into deeper sleep.

- Remember: You are getting "ping-ping-ping" constantly, 24/7.
- Best—turn ON the router only when you need it.
- Good—turn OFF the wireless router when you sleep.
- Use a $5 timer that you can buy at a hardware store to automatically turn OFF your router when you sleep and turn ON when you awake, or use remote control power switch.
- Before you turn OFF the router, ensure that the alarm system, landline telephone, any security or safety system, etc. do not go through the Router.

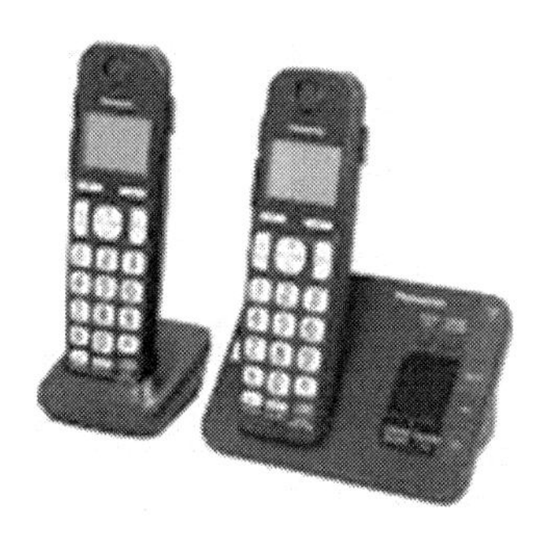

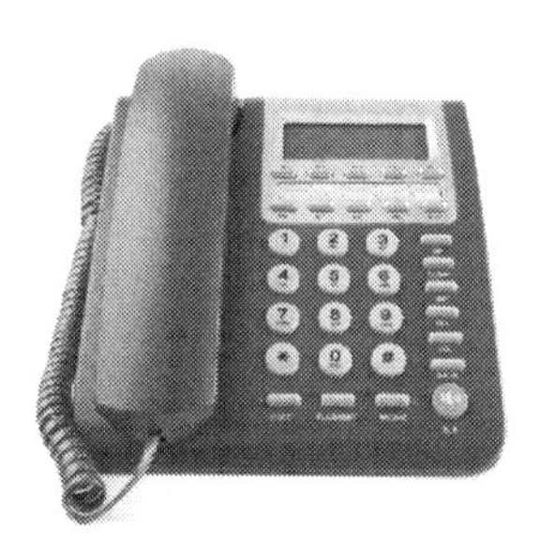

6. Go Retro!

Cordless Phones—just say NO!

Replace cordless phones with phones with cords that plug into wall jacks.

That's right, the old-fashioned corded phone.

- Cordless phones generate radiation just like a cell phone, when you're making a call.
- Cordless phone bases emit radiation even when you are NOT on a call.
- Don't use anything with a portable handset.

Would you allow a mini-cell tower in your home? That's exactly what the Cordless Phone Bases (DECT) simulate. They generate Radiation constantly, at extremely high levels—24/7—even when you are NOT making a call.

Story: Cancer on Your Nightstand

My wife was visiting some friends and found a cordless phone right on the gentleman's nightstand. I typically find them in an office or in a kitchen. Once in a while they are placed on a nightstand. This was just inches away from this man's pillow where he slept. And, sadly, he had multiple serious health issues involving his eyes and his heart and lungs, as well as cancer. Would you feel safe sleeping with a mini cell tower next to your head? Even if you tend to blame all or most diseases on your genetics, you might agree that it's not a good idea to "tempt" your genes. I'm talking common sense here.

When you replace your cordless phones with the old plug-in type, make sure there is no additional portable handset unit included. Those are wireless and that is what you are trying to avoid.

Example: John, a client with whom I was working, was so pleased that he had switched out his cordless phone with one that plugged in to the wall. But . . . it included an additional wireless handset. He had to return it for a REAL corded phone. These are available at most Big Box stores for around $25 without an answering machine, and about $35 with an answering machine. They work fine, and they do not emit radiation. And you can purchase one with a speaker mode so you can talk hands-free.

7. Read It Right!

Reading on a Laptop, iPad, Tablet, Kindle, Smartphone:

- All these devices are constantly trying to make a wireless, WiFi, or Bluetooth connection.
- This happens even if you are not actively searching, or downloading from the Internet. Ping – ping – ping – ping.

- To Stop the Radiation, such as when carrying a cell phone near your body, always keep Airplane Mode ON, and WiFi and Bluetooth OFF, when not using the device.
- Rather than streaming your books and games, download them, and enjoy them safely.
- Use on a DESK—unplugged, in battery mode. That way you avoid additional radiation from the wires. Also add or replace a wireless mouse and wireless keyboard with a wired USB mouse and a wired USB keyboard.
- Remember, you can't SEE the "ping-ping-ping" but it's there, 24/7, unless you turn it OFF. Also, if the device has a wireless, WiFi, and/or Bluetooth capability, you will need to put devices on a power strip and turn off the power strip (cut the power) when not in use. Some devices with wireless, WiFi, and/or Bluetooth capability still are producing radiation even if you turn the device off. And don't forget about surveillance—these devices can listen, locate, and log your personal and family information. Most smart devices are now designed to collect information when they are plugged in—some even if they are turned off. For more information on this, see They've Got Us Covered in Chapter 1.

Don't do this.

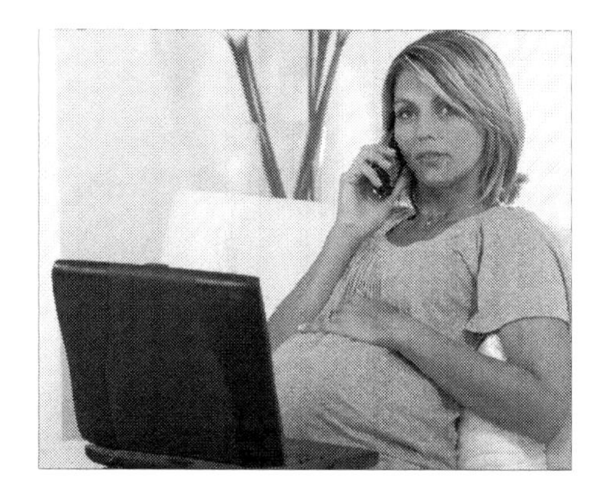

Do this—place the laptop on a table in battery mode, as far away as possible. And use a corded phone.

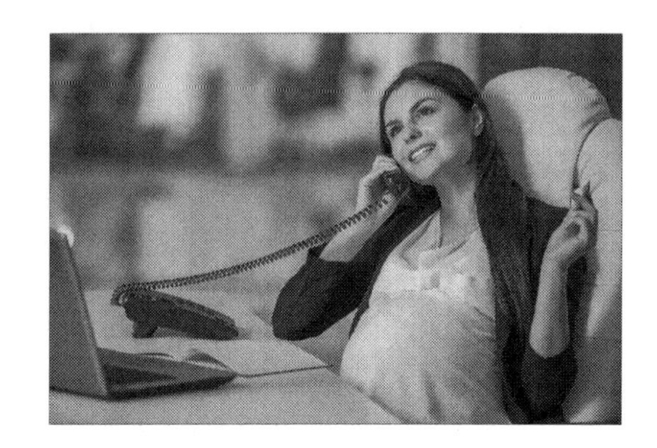

Story: Abdominal Cancer

One year at a Thanksgiving dinner I spoke with a young man in his early 30s who had just undergone abdominal surgery for a huge tumor. Thankfully, he had it successfully removed.

He asked me, "Do you think it could have had anything to do with my tablet?" I asked him how he used it. He told me he customarily read from his tablet while in bed every night for two to three hours. I was happy to instruct him on the safer use of tablets, and how I did my reading (and listening) on electronic devices safely by turning off the radiation. Regrettably, he went through a lot of suffering that possibly could have been avoided.

I like to listen to audible books on my phone while I walk. I simply download them, turn the radiation OFF, and enjoy the book radiation-free.

Airplane Mode ON + WiFi and Bluetooth OFF = Zero Radiation

Another story: I know a young man, Kevin, father of two small children, who listens to podcasts every night while in bed, with his phone on his stomach. And he sleeps with his phone on his stomach, well into the night.

I asked his wife whether he turned off the radiation. Since she didn't know, I asked her if he was able to receive calls during the night. She said yes. Maybe you can guess what I said to her –

If Kevin is able to receive a phone call, then he has not turned off the radiation and is listening to the podcasts in a highly unsafe mode. You can bet that Kevin got an earful from his wife when she returned home.

Kevin is not going to keel over dead this week or in the coming months. But what is he exposing himself to? And how long will it take to manifest itself? What are his genetic tendencies and exposure to other carcinogens? I know and love this young man. I'm planning on gifting him a copy of this book and hoping that he will take a more safe and healthy approach to using his electronic devices.

8. Better Off than Sorry

Electronic Devices

Printers, iPads, Tablets, Kindles, Laptops, Virtual-Reality Goggles, Smart home devices, and Computers can connect thru WiFi or Bluetooth.

- Turn these OFF when not using them, and get them as far away from you as possible. I recommend never using wireless Virtual-Augmented and Virtual-Reality Goggles.
- These devices generate radiation even in "Standby" mode. That's right. We sometimes think that just because our office equipment is "asleep" that it's not a problem. That's not true. And I can prove it by a simple measurement with the right kind of meter. The meter lights up like a Christmas tree, even when the device is dark. Ping-ping-ping-ping-ping. Communication from computer to printer can be hard wired via USB cable or as part of a network.

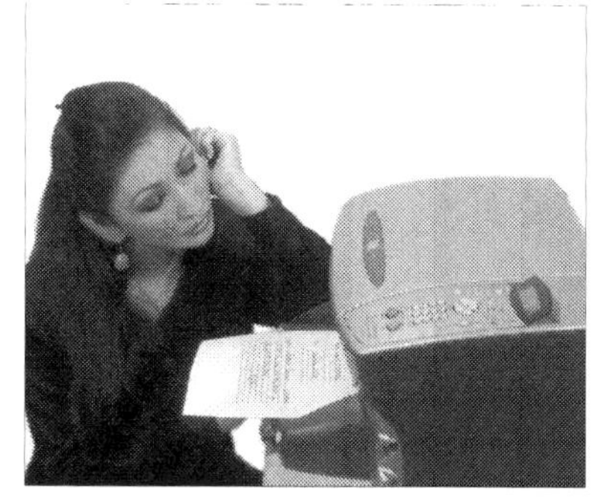

Watching a printer is tantamount to watching your food get zapped in a microwave. Step awaaaaaay. Let it goooooooooo.

9. Blueteeth?

Bluetooth devices are extremely dangerous.

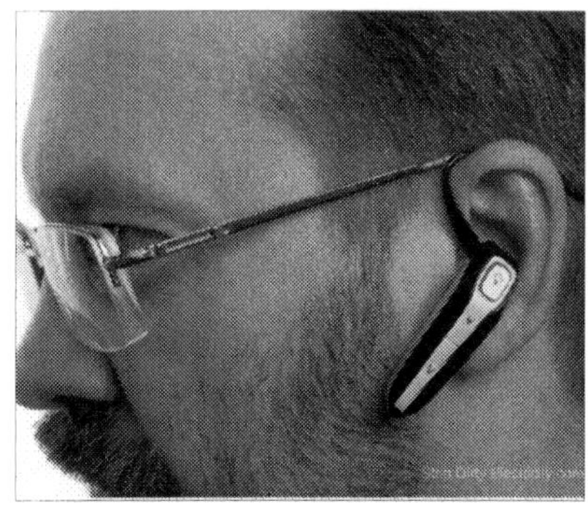

- They generate a high-level Wireless Radiation.
- They include: Ear Pieces, Cell Phone Watches, Wireless Headphones, Wireless Keyboards, Wireless Mouse, Fitness Watches/ Armbands, Smart Watches.
- If practical, never use a Bluetooth Ear piece or Wireless Headphones, or minimize its use.
- Fitness Watches/Armbands: I recommend that you don't use them. But if you do, use only when working out. That way, you limit your exposure to an hour or so, instead of 24/7.

Think of the rash of cancers above the neck—thyroid, salivary gland, throat cancer, brain tumors. Do you really want additional exposure to radiation around this part of your body?

Story: Bluetooth Melanoma

One day while at my chiropractor's office, he told me that one of his patients had developed melanoma—right under her Bluetooth ear piece. She was wondering if her Bluetooth device could have caused her melanoma.

Although I cannot say for certain what caused her cancer, I can say that we have never measured a Bluetooth ear piece that was not off-the-charts in radiation.

10. It's "Smarter" than You Think!

Smart Meter: A smart meter is an electronic utility meter that records consumption of electric energy and communicates that information back to the utility company for monitoring and billing. These meters are off-the-charts problematic on a number of levels.

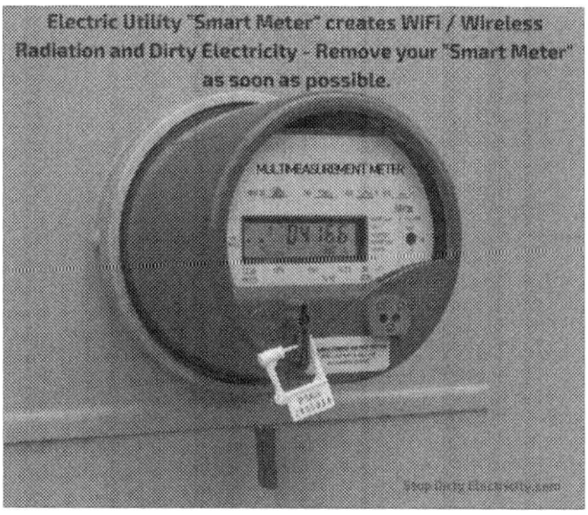

- Do you have a "smart meter"? Look for a digital display.
- Radiation levels can be up to 70 times stronger than a cell phone.
- Produce Wireless Radiation AND Dirty Electricity.
- Most Solar Panels require an additional Smart Meter to sell electricity back to the electrical utility company. (These need to be checked for radiation by a Certified Electro-magnetic Radiation Specialist.)
- Contact your Electric Utility Company and ask about its "Opt Out" Program.
- Replace ASAP with original meter—analog (the old kind that has the rotating dial).

Check out the "Take Back Your Power" documentary film directed by Josh del Sol: takebackyourpower.net. My wife calls this a horror movie. Thankfully, it is disturbing enough to elicit change in some people.

And just for FUN, watch this short video, "Smart Attack": tinyurl.com/ExposedSmartAttack.

Story: Hair Loss

I measured a house for EMR and suggested that the couple replace their "Smart Meter" with the old analog meter. The Smart Meter was located near their bedroom. They were fortunate to live in a location that had an "opt-out" program.

A couple of months later, the woman called and said, "My hair stopped falling out."

Hmmm. I didn't even know it ever was falling out. She said her hair had been falling out in clumps. I asked her to go back and look at her records to determine when it started falling out.

She concluded that it started falling out shortly after the Smart Meter had been installed.

Clearly, this does not happen to everyone, or there would be a run on wigs, and beauty salons would be closing right and left. But the Smart Meter seemed to be a fright factor to this particular woman's hair health. Thankfully, it completely reversed once the offending digital smart meter was replaced.

11. BONUS: We've Got You Covered, Baby!

Baby Monitors: Ooooh, they are so convenient. And everybody's using them.

Think about it. A monitor is often placed right at the baby's head, and, often, right at a parent's head as well.

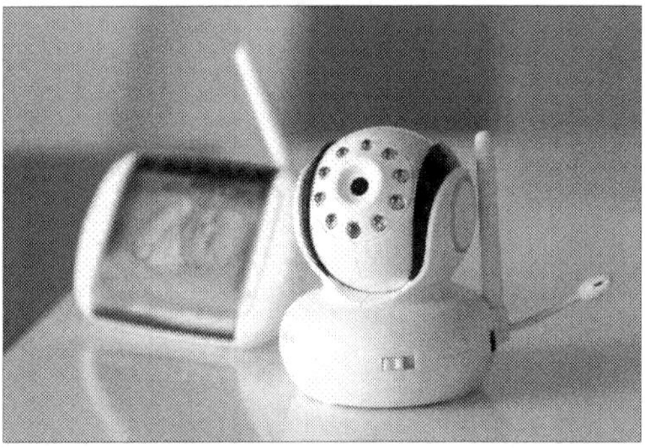

- Baby Monitors can generate Wireless, WiFi, or Bluetooth Radiation constantly. Ping-ping-ping-ping.
- Radiation is at Baby's Head and Parents' Unit.
- We recommend that you don't use one. But if using, place as far away as possible from the baby and the parents.
- You can measure it with a Safe and Sound Classic or an Acousticom 2 meter, or a similar meter, to identify a safer location.
- Some monitors are worse than others. You must measure them to be sure.
- There are baby monitors that are wired (non-WiFi). You will have to check for the three types of radiation from

wires (electric, magnetic, and dirty electricity). But this is probably a better option, if you must use one.

View a one-minute video at: Tinyurl.com/ExposedBaby.

I have heard so many disturbing stories of toddlers who develop autism, when, for a while, the children seemed to progress normally, then took a sudden turn for the worse. Could there be a link between exposure to radiation, which compromises the blood-brain barrier, so that dangerous chemicals or heavy metals seep into the brain? How many of these babies had a baby monitor at their heads? And is it worth the risk? (If you use a baby monitor, or know someone who does, this is a good time to review Chapter 1: What's It Doing to Our Children?)

I spoke with a young working mother of two who was interested in reducing the radiation in her home. I shared some of these suggestions and her response was, "I don't have time."

So, I asked her, "What if you took thirty days, and made one small, one-minute change each day?"

She thought about it . . . and affirmed, "Yeah, I can do that."

Actions for Today:

- ✓ Start today—implement as many of these suggestions as you can.
- ✓ Make a plan to make one small change every day for 30 days.
- ✓ Share with friends and family.

Need or want more solutions right now?

Go to Chapters 7 and 9 and Appendix I for your Comprehensive Home Safety Audit.

Chapter 9

But WAIT. There's MORE.

Now I Lay Me Down to Sleep

Creating a "sleep sanctuary" is one of the kindest acts you can do for yourself and your family, and even for your pets.

You may be familiar with these recommendations for improving sleep:

1. Keep it dark.
2. Shhhhh. Be still.
3. Cool but not cold. Or, if you prefer, warm but not hot.
4. Limit alcohol and caffeine in the evening hours.
5. Minimize the clutter in your bedroom.
6. Use natural fabrics in your bedding materials.
7. Make sure your bed and pillow are comfortable.
8. Try to maintain a regular sleep and waking schedule.
9. Keep pets off the bed. Sorry.
10. Try to relax your mind and wind down from the business of the day.
11. Be careful about prescription or herbal sleep inducers.
12. Include exercise as part of your daily routine, but not close to bedtime.

Let's add some EMR tips to your bedroom:

13. Get all electronics off of your nightstand. Move them as far away as possible or to another room. (Battery-operated clocks are OK.)
14. Limit screen time to daytime. The blue light itself

emanating from the screen, in addition to the EMR, interrupts sleep and decreases melatonin production.

15. Check to see whether the wall behind your pillow is where your breaker box is located, or some other electrical or electronic device. You may need to reposition your headboard to a more favorable location.
16. Use dirty electricity plug-in filters in the outlets in your bedroom. This may require a meter and consultation from a Certified Electromagnetic Radiation Specialist, as occasionally the magnetic fields will rise with the plug-in filters. (Please review Three Bits of Caution on page 182.)

Dirty Electricity Advanced Techniques:

Sometimes dirty electricity is harder to reduce, especially with solar panels, newer swimming pool pumps with variable speed motors, and also air conditioning and heating systems with variable speed motors.

If you find yourself in this situation you can:

- Check to see which outlet has the highest dirty electricity in your home.
- Start with that outlet.
- If the dirty electricity does not reduce to a reasonable level just plugging in filters into the wall outlets directly, then try a $4 power strip and plug the filters into the power strip. (Levels listed in Chapter 12)
- Re-measure the outlets in that room and reduce the next highest outlet in the room with the same techniques.
- Do these techniques throughout your home.

17. At night you can turn off circuit breakers to the bedrooms. Test it for several days and determine whether it enhances your sleep or not. Make sure smoke detectors, and safety and security systems, are not affected when breakers are being switched off. (And make sure you

don't turn off the switch that controls the refrigerator. I'm still hearing about that one from my wife.)

18. Turn off router at night. If you cannot remember to do this, get a $5 timer at big-box hardware stores so that it turns on and off automatically, or use a remote control power switch.
19. Remove electric blankets.
20. Get medical stuff, such as a CPAP machine or Nebulizer, as far away from your pillow as possible.
21. If you have an electric bed, unplug it when you sleep. Or, use a remote control switch to turn power to the bed off when you sleep. You can purchase a remote control shut-off switch. Cost? Less than $9.00.
22. Unplug any electric cords around your bed. Use a remote control switch to turn off power from the outlet when you sleep. You can purchase a remote control shut-off switch. Cost? Less than $9.00. If you need more outlets, plug a power strip into to the remote control switch.
23. Make your bedroom a low-tech zone.
24. If you are EHS—electromagnetic hypersensitive—you may want to turn off breakers and explore different shielding options. Make sure smoke detectors, and safety and security systems, are not affected when breakers are being switched off. Shielding is sometimes tricky, so you need to consult a Certified Electromagnetic Radiation Specialist, or at least have your own meters. If you do use shielding, you must measure before the shielding is installed and then after the shielding is installed to verify that the radiation levels did not increase. You must measure all four types of radiation. (See Chapter 12 for the "Concern" levels of radiation.)

Sleep in heavenly peace. Zzzzzzz.

Trains, Planes and Automobiles

We all do it. Check one last email as the plane begins taxiing down the runway. Catch up on phone calls while driving or riding the subway. Good use of your time, right?

When using a cell phone in what is essentially a metal box traveling at a fast speed, your phone is working all the harder to connect. It produces even more radiation. So, instead of ping-ping-ping, your phone is going pingpingpingpingpingpingping.

The same holds true for an elevator. Just waiting until you reach your floor destination can save you an unwanted, extra-high dose of radiation. And spare you the annoying looks of the captive audience in that enclosed space.

Bars are important. (Not the kind for drinking.) When traveling, you may lose bars, and that means, once again, that your phone is working harder to deliver your communication. That means more radiation is coming your way. Much smarter to just wait a few minutes until your reception improves. And there is less chance of dropping a call.

Travel wisely.

Cars

They are now all equipped with hands-free Bluetooth devices. Admittedly, it's probably safer than juggling a phone in your hand, on your shoulder, or to your ear—in some states, it's the law. And the steering wheel controls and voice-activated systems are slick. But there are problems with hands-free as well.

First of all, there is the obvious—constant exposure to Wireless/WiFi/Bluetooth radiation. Not a problem if you don't spend a lot of time driving. But what about those long road trips? Or sales reps who must drive around all day, every day?

I use a portable Bluetooth device that clips onto my visor. I can turn it on and off as needed, thus limiting my exposure on long road trips. It works OK. But most new cars don't have that option. (Good reason to keep your old car running.) In most newer cars, the Bluetooth function is on, whether you are using it on a phone call or not. There are ways to disable that. You might need to call the car manufacturer or your local car dealer to find out how to disable the Bluetooth feature.

Some people who are highly sensitive to EMR have gone to great lengths to custom design their vehicles with their own hands-free calling systems using exterior antennas. Good for them!

Additionally, there is a lot of concern about distracted driving. Some suggest that hands-free phone use isn't much safer than hand-held. Talking on the phone in any mode is still distracted driving.

I remember when I bought my first cell phone. It was a flip phone. It was purely for emergency use, to make urgent out-going calls. I kept the phone in the glove compartment and turned off. How things have changed. How did we get so busy that we depend on our phones almost every minute of every day?

What about GPS? I still use one of the old portable GPS devices that plug into the cigarette lighter and mount on the window. They work OK. Also, it is possible to use the GPS on your phone while still cutting off the radiation. Here's how:

1. Connect to your destination as you would normally do.

2. After you connect and get directions, turn airplane mode ON, and WiFi and Bluetooth OFF.

On my particular phone, I get a modified version of GPS. The map comes up and the voice tells me to turn, but it might not state the name of the roadway. Also, it does not automatically re-route with voice commands if I miss a turn, nor does it give live traffic updates or road conditions. But it is still usable, without radiation exposure. You will have to test this out on your own phone to see whether it is usable for your needs.

I got the idea from the book *The Non-Tinfoil Guide to EMFs—How to Fix Our Stupid Use of Technology* by Nicolas Pineault (2017). He tried it on an iPhone 6. And I tested the GPS on my Android Samsung Galaxy smartphone. It did work, but it limited some of the phones' functions.

Try not to use your phone in a moving metal box.

Electric Cars

A colleague and I test drove several electric cars at the AltCar Expo & Conference in Santa Monica, California. While he drove, I measured. I tested for electric and magnetic radiation. The electric and magnetic radiation was very high in some of the vehicles. This colleague had a client who had to return her electric car because she could not tolerate the radiation from her particular model. The bottom line is that all the cars had higher electro-pollution, and some were worse than others. Or should I say, some were better than others. As in most cases, you must measure to be sure.

DIM—Do It MySELF

Retro is in vogue. Blast-from-the-past fashion and musical groups are so popular! So let's add to the list:

- ✓ Go back to battery-operated clocks and devices, where possible.
- ✓ Corded phones are the way to go.
- ✓ Return to the wired mouse and wired keyboard for your computer. They are very inexpensive. As an extra safety precaution, take the batteries out of the wireless mouse and wireless keyboard, as they can sometimes continue to transmit even when they are not being used.
- ✓ Hard wire your printer, but you will still need to turn off the WiFi/Bluetooth on the printer, if you can't or don't want to turn off the device.
- ✓ Take your computer back to hard-wired Ethernet. It's faster anyway. And more secure. I worked with a couple where the husband was resistant to hard wiring his computer. But his wife urged him to do that. Once installed, he had a much faster and more secure connection to the Internet. Happy wife, happy life.
- ✓ Resist the latest WiFi gadgets. You might not need them.

- ✓ Screw in the old-fashioned light bulbs, or use halogen bulbs with the wide, screw-in base.
- ✓ Opt out of the "Smart Meter" Digital Electric Utility Meter and go back to the original analog utility meter and the "meter man."

What do you want me to do? Regress? Sort of. Start living in the past using batteries and cords instead of WiFi/Bluetooth whenever possible. And the old-fashioned phones and light bulbs produce no EMR.

"Some of the most mundane devices are designed to accomplish a simple task extremely well—and in some cases they still execute those duties better than their high-tech brethren," says Brian X. Chen, the *New York Times*' lead consumer technology reporter. (Chen, 2018)

Take Control—Right Now

There are so many wireless items over which you can take control—right now. But electrical cords and wiring in your walls also have issues, creating electric and magnetic radiation, and dirty electricity.

The good news is that there are some DIM/DIY actions that will bump up your success—BAM!

I gave you some in-a-nutshell, rule-of-thumb fixes for radiation traveling on wires in Chapter 7, and please review the Three Bits of Caution on page 178. Fixes for radiation through the air were in Chapter 8. If you're motivated to advance to the next level and really be sure that what you are doing is having its intended effect, you need to learn how to use a meter.

If you do not have a Certified Electromagnetic Radiation Specialist in your area, there is another option. On my website are DIY Master Class Video Packages that take you through every room in your house. The videos are two to four minutes long and demonstrate:

- ➢ What meter to use.
- ➢ How to measure.

- ➢ What and where to measure.
- ➢ What the results mean.
- ➢ The levels of "concern."
- ➢ How to remediate.
- ➢ Test and verify.

A sample of the videos can be found at YouTube: Stop Dirty Electricity, and at Facebook: StopDirtyElectricity. I think you will agree that the DIY videos are easy to follow. And when you purchase an online DIY Master Class Video Package, it entitles you to a free phone or email consultation.

Chapter 11 tells you HOW to use the meters. And the use of the meters is also covered in the videos.

Yes, you can do it yourself.

Chapter 12 tells you what numbers to look for to keep you, your family, and your pets as safe as possible from radiation.

Appendix I provides a comprehensive safety audit of every room in your house with every possible gadget and gizmo you could possibly own. It is complete and up-to-date, as of my most recent visit to the annual Consumer Electronics Show. The list will be updated every year on my website.

So, how do you DIY?

- ✓ Use the knowledge and tools I have included in this book.
- ✓ Purchase the three meters I have recommended. (If you already own different meters, they may still be usable. You will need to consult a Certified Electromagnetic Radiation Specialist to determine whether the meters are of sufficient quality and sensitivity to be used and to assess measurement units and conversions.
- ✓ Subscribe to the DIY Master Class Video Program on my website for step-by-step instructions. Or, send me an email at: bill@stopdirtyelecticity.com, and I can get you started.
- ✓ Please consult a Certified Electromagnetic Radiation Specialist in your area for assistance before launching your DIY program—if at all possible.

What a great family or group project this would be to join forces and tackle the EMR together. You could share the knowledge, experience, and cost, and really help those you care about most. There is a lot YOU can do.

Say it out loud—I can DIM. I can Do It Myself.

EMF Rescue

Leave no wire untapped—call the "House Doctor."

How serious is this? If one of your water pipes were leaking, you could see evidence in your wall or ceiling. You would call a plumber ASAP to repair the issue and prevent further damage.

But have you thought about calling a "House Doctor" to check for electrical "leakage"? You can't see it, feel it, taste it, or smell it. But electricity could be "leaking" from the wires and cables in your home.

When you are sick, how do you know when it's time to call the doctor? You have unanswered symptoms and questions. You need access to more sophisticated diagnostics. You need to tap in to the doctor's experience and the art as well as the science.

You've heard of "Ghost Busters." Well, I'm kind of a "House Doctor," sweeping away invisible, harmful radiation. The solutions are scientific and measurable. And now is the time to take control of this growing menace to your health.

Also, wireless poisoning is gaining headline attention. But very few people are aware of the potential danger of radiation exposure from the wiring in their homes.

There is a LOT you can do on your own to reduce your exposure to harmful EMR. Most of the solutions in this section are easily and immediately implemented by almost anyone. And most of these remedies are free. Additionally, you can purchase an online DIY Master Class Video Package to refine and increase your effectiveness, and to test and verify the results. Go to StopDirtyElectricity.com and get started.

Why Do I Need a Specialist?

So, what can a Certified Electromagnetic Radiation Specialist offer that you cannot already do? Difficult situations require advanced diagnostics and artful remediation using expensive, high-end meters to verify results:

EMF from the outside—there are things outside of our control on the outside of our homes, such as a neighbor who won't get rid of his smart meter, a cell tower on the hillside, dirty electricity entering our homes from a power substation, high-voltage wires in our backyards. Shielding and/or special paint may need to be considered.

Windows—these can be tricky. Sometimes when shielding is applied, radiation actually enters a room through a window and bounces around inside the room. You need a trained Certified EMR Specialist to know what to look for.

Solar Power—this must be carefully measured for dirty electricity and wireless radiation from a smart meter. This takes time and employs the art and science that come from advanced training and experience in order to remedy.

Dirty electricity riding on electrical cables can come from outside the home and can be difficult to track down.

Reducing the dirty electricity with the use of filters—this takes time to go back and forth between outlets, testing the effect of dirty electricity filters on the other types of radiation. Sometimes, you can lower one type of radiation while increasing another type. Experience and knowledge is important. Please review Dirty Electricity Advanced Techniques on page 174.

Three Bits of Caution:

1. Dirty electricity filters effectively lower dirty electricity. But on occasion they can raise magnetic fields. You have to check and double check. If this happens, consult a Certified EMR Specialist for remediation.
2. There are some electromagnetic hypersensitive people who react better with one filter or the other. If you are

EHS, you may want to compare how you feel with both filters and determine which one works best for you. Test them out. If you have a negative reaction, pull them out and try the other type of filter. If neither is right for you, there are other filter options for EHS people, but they are more expensive. Greenwave has a different type of filter that some EHS people seem to do better with, at the same price.

3. It rarely happens, but if you do feel worse when you plug in dirty electricity filters, remove them and call either a Certified Electromagnetic Radiation Specialist or the manufacturer of the filter for remediation.

Faulty Wiring—there are times when an EMR-aware electrician must be employed to work with your Certified Electromagnetic Radiation Specialist to detect and remediate wiring errors.

Saunas—takes time and problem solving. Some that claim to be "Low EMF" are low in only one of the four types of radiation. I tested one recently and found only one spot to sit where it was free of ALL four types of radiation. Whew! I was sweating, and the sauna wasn't even turned on.

Buyer Beware—there are people claiming to rid your home of radiation whose qualifications and experience are limited. They often use low-cost, ineffective meters. Or, they are testing for only one or two types of radiation.

Remember, there is radiation that travels through the AIR. And there are three different types that radiate from WIRES. All are potentially damaging to your health.

Regrettably, some people have acquired a false sense of security, thinking that they are safe from radiation, when they really are not safe at all.

A Certified Electromagnetic Radiation Specialist is often able to reduce most types of EMR by more than 90 percent in a single-family, detached home. And all remedies can be measured, verified, and repeated.

Apartments, condos, townhomes and interior office spaces are a different story. They can be surrounded on all sides as well as above and below. So the bombardment and saturation from neighboring spaces can be extreme. What's really bad is when you find an entire bank of smart meters on a wall where your living space is located. Still, there are solutions we can apply to help you reduce your exposure. In all cases, we strive for ALARA (As Low As Reasonably Achievable).

I hope this section, EMR Rescue, doesn't discourage you from DIM/DIY action. There is a LOT you can do today with the right information and tools. Phone consultation with an expert is always an option if you run into problems. But there are times when you do need to call the House Doctor.

To find a Certified Electromagnetic Radiation Specialist in your area, go to the Building Biology Institute website: hbelc.org/find-an-expert.

Actions for Today:

- ✓ Make your sleeping area a priority.
- ✓ Limit your cell phone use while traveling in a car, train, or riding in an elevator.
- ✓ Consider starting the DIY Master Class Video Program with a free phone or email consultation to help lower harmful radiation in your home or work space and have the ability to also help family and friends. For more information, visit my website: StopDirtyElectricity.com.
- ✓ Or make an appointment with a Certified Electromagnetic Radiation Specialist to do an EMF Home Inspection.

Need or want more solutions right now?

Go to Chapters 7 and 8 and Appendix I for your Comprehensive Home Safety Audit.

SECTION III

What About?
FAQ

Chapter 10

What About Shielding Cases, Decals, Dots, and Crystals?

What's worse than having an unsafe exposure? Having a FALSE sense of security.

Shielding Cases

Many people tell me they don't worry about excessive cell phone use because they have purchased a shielding case.

So, I ask to test it. I test all six sides—top, bottom, left, right, front, back. I test with the phone on, but not in use. I test with the phone in use, with Wireless/WiFi/Bluetooth on. Invariably, the phone will measure low radiation, and the owner will smugly nod . . . until I get to the LEAK-out side or sides. You see, IF you are able to make and receive calls and data, the Wireless/WiFi/Bluetooth signal has to go in and out SOMEwhere.

Think about it. If you put your phone in a totally shielded case, it would cut out ALL Wireless/WiFi/Bluetooth signals, and therefore would be non-functional. This would apply to tablets, iPads, Kindles, and laptop shields as well. While they may prevent EMR from radiating out onto your lap, just because you have a shielding case does not automatically mean you are safe. How about your torso, neck, and head? My recommendation is that you take the precautions detailed earlier and not rely completely on a shielding case to protect you.

Decals and Dots

Another common misunderstanding about preventing cell phone and tablet radiation is the use of special decals and dots on the back of the phone that claim to modify or absorb the radiation. People tell me someone measured the radiation with a meter and "proved" that the radiation was lowered when the sticker was placed on the phone. Sadly, the meter used is almost always an inexpensive meter that measures magnetic radiation.

It can be the wrong meter,
measuring the wrong thing.

It isn't even measuring the offense of wireless radiation. And, yes, the dots and decals sometimes show a lowering of magnetic radiation. But that really is not the major issue of cell phones and tablets. What Certified Electromagnetic Radiation Specialists do is scientific and measurable. But one must have the right science and the right measurement devices that measure all four types of EMR.

Crystals and Pendants

This is a difficult one, as it gets into "body energy fields." That is not my area of expertise. I can only say that the cell phones I have tested, where the owner was wearing a crystal that protected him or her from Wireless/WiFi/Bluetooth, were still emitting dangerous levels of radiation. The claim is that the body itself is impervious to the incoming radiation. Some people feel better when wearing a crystal or pendant. But that is something I cannot test and verify. I recommend that you always reduce all four types of radiation first, and that includes radiation traveling through the air and from the wires.

Grounding Pads and Earthing

These items must be tested to prove their efficacy. There are some people who say they feel better using these things. However, all types of radiation, Wireless/WiFi/Bluetooth radiation, Electric radiation, magnetic radiation, and dirty electricity, must still be lowered. Grounding is not a sure thing. One thing to consider is that ground currents sometimes change in a particular location, so an annual measurement at the location of your grounding stake, or at the grounding point inside the home, is recommended.

Shielded Clothing

Some shielded clothing does work. People who are EMR sensitive have gotten relief of their symptoms AND there can be a measurable verification by reputable EMR specialists using top-of-the-line meters.

However, I cannot attest to the fashion statement thereof. OK. To be fair, I have seen some decent-looking wearables that were made of shielding materials. And, with the implementation of 5G and IoT, I may have to reconsider.

Out of Africa:

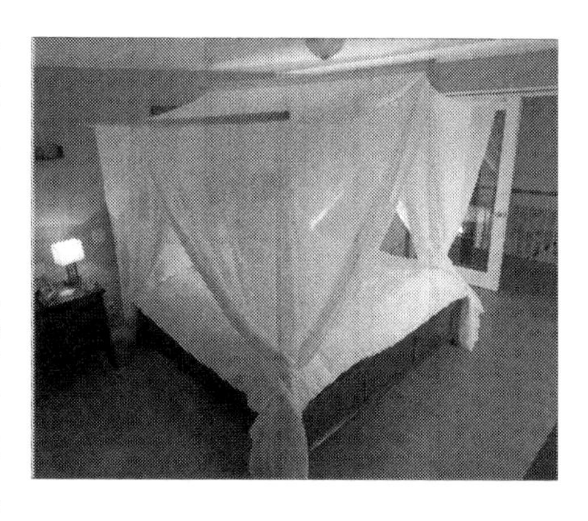

There is a specially manufactured canopy-style tent that drapes over a frame and shields your bed from WiFi/Wireless/Bluetooth radiation. It is particularly useful when there are outside sources of radiation that cannot be controlled by the home owner. It does work and can be measured and verified. And it's kind of cool looking. It's available at Safe Living Technologies: slt.co. For 5% off, use coupon code safe7 at checkout.

If your bedroom is on the second floor or higher, be sure you put protective shielding underneath the bed as well. This ensures that radiation will not come through the floor and be trapped inside the canopy.

Oils

Yes, you read correctly. Oils. I've had people bring their phones to me and say that their phones were rubbed with a special EMR repellent oil. They anoint their phones with oil every few days to keep safe from radiation. Are they safe from radiation? If you have been paying attention, you will know what I am about to say. One must meticulously measure using the right meters, and know what to look for. I've never measured an "oil'd" phone that was safe. I believe in the healing properties of oils for people, but have not found oil to be effective for phones.

The Building Biology Institute does address some of these items. This is the body of experts that certifies Electromagnetic Radiation Specialists, such as myself. We acknowledge that there are thousands of EHS people who have gotten some measure of relief by the above devices. Additionally, there is some evidence of biological response shown in live-blood analysis and thermography.

However, readings on our professional, carefully calibrated meters are not altered with the use of pendants, crystals, home harmonizers, etc. So, we advise caution to not use "subtle energy devices" as the first or sole means of protection. We encourage reduction/elimination strategies that are measurable in a consistent manner. We think it is best to identify and reduce sources of EMFs in the first place, rather than attempting to merely "neutralize" their effects.

For additional information, see "Subtle Energy Devices: An IBE Position Paper": https://buildingbiologyinstitute.org/free-downloads/.

FAQ

Dimmer Switches

Do I really have to get rid of them? You say, "I love my mood lights, and I'm not going to give them up."

OK. Just use it sparingly, and turn the switch completely OFF when you are not in the mood. But if you are highly sensitive to EMF, you may want to change dimmers to regular switches.

Electric Blankets

Do I have to give up my cozy comfort?

Sorry, I have never measured one that was in the safe range. Go back to goose down or an old-fashioned quilt.

I have measured electric blankets that were more than 500 times the "No Concern" level.

Light Bulbs

What about those energy-saving light bulbs?

Ooooh, yeah. Fluorescent lights, CFL bulbs. Dispose of them safely and replace with incandescent bulbs. Halogen are OK as long as they have the wide base and screw into the socket—they do not emit radiation.

I have found that most LEDs create dirty electricity—and they also flicker, which can be hard on your eyes. Additionally, the blue light quality suppresses melatonin production if you use them before you go to sleep. The original incandescent light bulbs that have been around for 100 years work well and do not emit radiation.

Batteries

What about DC batteries?

They are safe for most people. Some EHS people react to them.

Electronic Medical Devices

There are some medical devices that use electrical pulses to stimulate bone growth and nerve repair. I know, because my wife used these therapies during physical therapy after a cycling accident. I think using therapeutic electrical stimulation for a specific purpose for a limited time is OK. There are many other medical treatments using electricity, but this isn't what this book is about. You have to weigh the risks and benefits, and consult with your physician.

Shielding Paint

There is specially designed paint that can be used to shield your home, inside or outside, from radiation through the AIR and electric radiation. It is black. Yes, black. And must be carefully applied using a designated pattern, one horizontal coat of paint and one vertical coat of paint is best. After two coats of black paint, your preferred color may take as much as two to three coats, depending on the color. Also, depending on the material out of which your house is made, it may require more paint. (Stucco, for example, is porous and may require more paint.)

I learned recently that a new cell tower could be installed just three blocks from our home. Can we oppose it? Probably not. I'm planning on painting the exterior portion of my house that faces the cell tower and to add some shielding in the attic or on the roof. At least I'll be ready for 5G. I will take EMR/EMF measurements before and after. I might have to radiation-proof that wall of my home. That's much easier than trying to fight city hall.

The placement has to be approved by the local governing body. However, if you or your neighbors appeal the placement of a cell tower near your homes, remember that, under the current federal telecommunications legislation, placement of a cell tower can never be denied because of health concerns or environmental concerns.

As 5G legislation is being brought forward, cell phone companies are now trying to remove the local governing body's approval so that only the FCC would have the power to deny a cell phone tower placement. Good luck in trying to get the FCC to deny a placement, keeping in mind it cannot be denied for health or environmental concerns.

Shielding Window Film

This is effective. If you paint the walls, the next place you have to shield are the windows. I'm planning on using it on my own house, if I paint it. It is always necessary to consult a Certified Electromagnetic Radiation Specialist with calibrated meters to measure before and after.

A Word of Caution

Shielding is always tricky. If there are any "chinks in the armor," radiation can actually get trapped and bounce around inside. There are many factors to consider, so it's always necessary to consult a Certified EMR Specialist who can measure before-and-after results.

Undoubtedly, there are other devices and techniques out there that I have not encountered. And new ones will be developed.

The only way to be sure that you are reducing your radiation is to measure all four types of radiation. And, in doing this,

✓ Know what you are doing.
✓ Think through the mechanics of the claims of the product.
✓ Implement the EMR-reducing techniques presented in this book.
✓ Use the correct equipment if you do your own metering.
✓ Know the "Concern" levels listed in Chapter 12.
✓ Know how to remediate.
✓ Consult with a Certified EMR Specialist.

This book gives you the KNOWLEDGE to do most of this for little or no cost at all. Many of these shielding items can be purchased at Safe Living Technologies: slt.co. For an additional 5% off, use coupon code safe7 at checkout.

Actions for Today:

- ✓ Carefully measure with the correct meter(s) before you buy a device and entrust your health to it.
- ✓ Replace energy-saving light bulbs with incandescent or halogen (only with the wide, screw-in base).
- ✓ Consider some shielding options, if no other options are available.
- ✓ Use common sense and sales resistance when it comes to fairy dust.

Need or want solutions right now?

Go to Chapters 7, 8 and 9 (more than 30 pages of solutions) and Appendix I for your Comprehensive Home Safety Audit.

Chapter 11

Meter, Meter, on the Wall . . .

Not All Meters Are Created Equal

There are meters. And then there are meters. Not all meters are created equal.

The measuring devices we use and recommend are high-quality residential meters that have been cross-referenced with professionally calibrated meters. They are reliable and surprisingly easy to use.

Regrettably, some people are using meters that are not sensitive enough to detect levels of radiation within the appropriate "Concern" levels. If you already have meters, you might want to compare your ranges with the "Concern" levels listed in the next chapter.

The meters I recommend are affordable, especially if a few friends and/or family members agree to go in together on them. It could be a cool community or family project—to learn about and remediate the radiation in your living spaces, work areas, and, most importantly, your sleeping areas.

The three types of meters you need to measure all four types of radiation (through the AIR and from the WIRES) are:

1. Safe and Sound Classic or Acousticom 2— WiFi/ Wireless/Bluetooth/RF Radiation
2. Gigahertz ME3030B—magnetic radiation AND electric radiation
3. Greenwave Meter or Stetzer Meter—dirty electricity

Note: Dirty electricity is the only type of radiation for which there are filters that will reduce radiation. I recommend Greenwave Filters or Stetzer Filters. Please review Three Bits of Caution on page 178.

Meter Details

To measure radiation through the AIR:

WiFi/Wireless/Bluetooth/RF/Microwave Radiation

Safe and Sound Classic

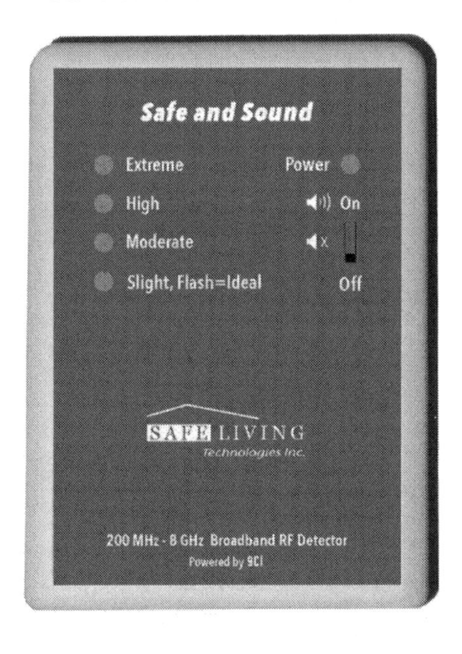

Acousticom 2

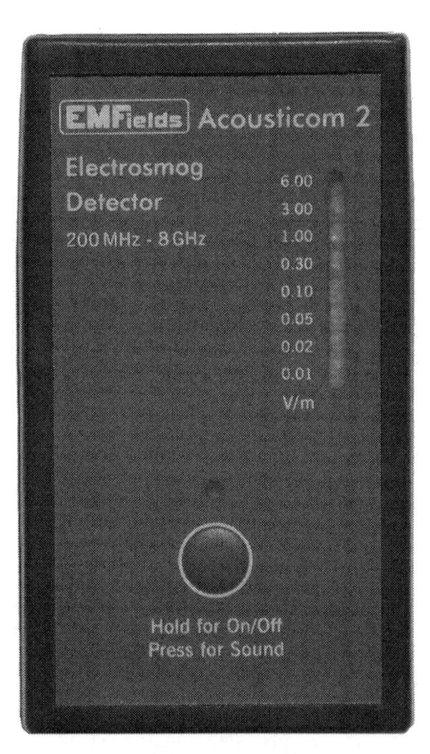

These are great little meters. They are easy to use and very affordable.

The Safe and Sound Classic shows, with LED lights, Extreme, High, Moderate, or Slight concern.

With Acousticom 2, check the lights and numbers for the appropriate level of "Concern" listed in Chapter 12.

Both meters are quite accurate and easy to carry. An audible tone similar to that of a Geiger counter indicates the level of exposure. They are the size of a deck of cards. They're a big hit at a party!

Just use the ON button and you are ready to go. Hold the meter near a Wireless, WiFi, or Bluetooth device, such as a cell phone or tablet or router, or the dreaded microwave oven.

Distance is your friend. If radiation is detected, step away from the device. Or turn it OFF at the source.

To measure radiation coming from WIRES, two different meters are used:

Measuring Electric Radiation AND Magnetic Radiation

Gigahertz ME3030B

This is an exceptional Entry-level Meter.

- Easy to Operate: simply power on the unit, select mode of operation, "E" for Electric field or "M" for Magnetic field, then scan the area of concern.
- LCD digital display will indicate the total field strength of all sources within its frequency range.

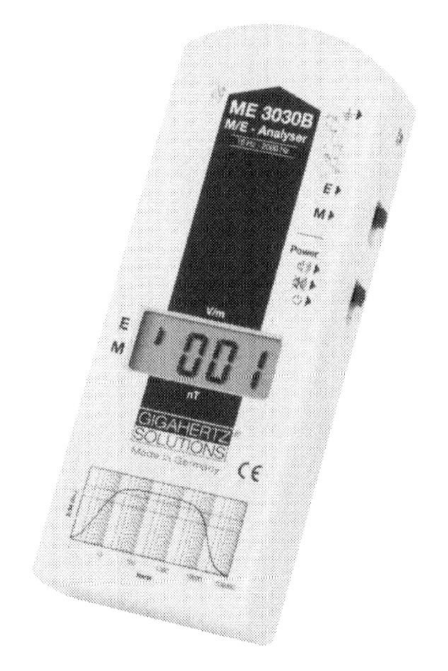

- Audible tone similar to that of a Geiger counter indicates level of exposure.
- Excellent sensitivity: able to accurately identify electric fields down to 1 V/m and magnetic fields to 1 nT. (Don't be intimidated by the numbers and units. I provide easy-to-interpret "Concern" levels for all meters.)
- Readings are 98 percent accurate within the 16 Hertz to 2000 Hertz frequency range. Sources of radiation in this

range include all standard household appliances, electronic devices, electrical wiring and wiring errors, high-voltage power lines, and electrical power transformers.
- Powered by a 9V alkaline battery (included).
- All Gigahertz Solutions meters are backed by a two-year manufacturer's warranty.

Please note: When using this meter for testing for electric fields, you must set the meter down and step away three or four feet, otherwise your body will act as an antenna and cause a false reading. This does not happen when measuring for magnetic fields.

To obtain any of these three meters, go to: Safe Living Technologies at slt.co. For 5% off, use coupon code safe7 at checkout.

Measuring Dirty Electricity

There are two manufacturers that I recommend:

Greenwave Dirty Electricity Meter

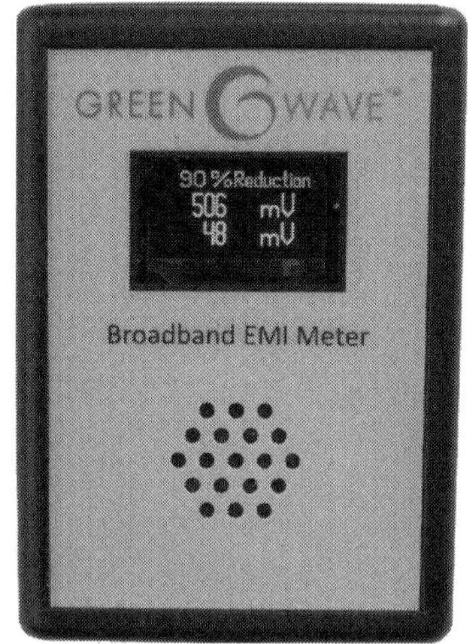

This basic, easy-to-use meter measures the amount of dirty electricity (high-frequency voltage transients and harmonics) present on the wiring in buildings. Find out the level of electrical pollution on your wiring at home, work, etc. Compatible with 50/60-Hz electrical circuits with voltage anywhere between 100V and 240V. It comes with a plug suitable for the electrical outlets in your environment.

To purchase online, go to the Greenwave website: greenwavefilters.com. For 5% off, use coupon code safe7 at checkout.

Before you use any filters, please review Three Bits of Caution on page 182.

Plug the meter into a wall outlet and read the number. If you have high levels of dirty electricity, plug in a filter. Take the reading again. You should see a dramatic drop into the safe level. However, in rare cases it may take two filters. Also, try placing a second filter in a different outlet near the one you are testing. That may make a difference. Please review Dirty Electricity Advanced Techniques on page 174.

Stetzer Dirty Electricity Meter

The Stetzer has an easy-to-use digital display that shows you the amount of dirty electricity present on an electrical circuit in your home or office.

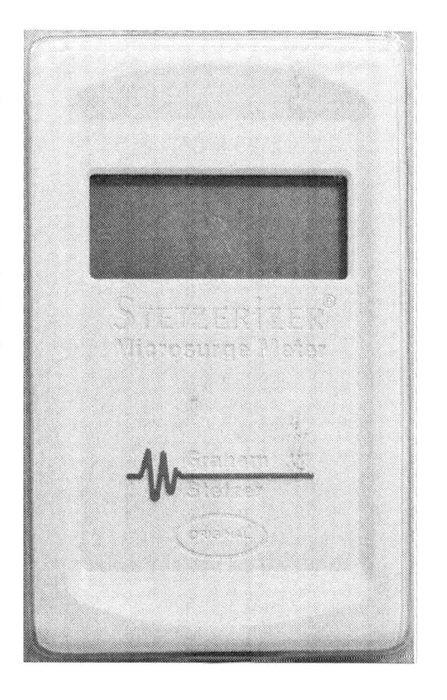

The GS meter measures the level of harmful electromagnetic "energy" present, and its primary use is to help with effective filter installation. Microsurge meters are low-cost and easy to use by non-technical people. The meters were designed to measure radio-frequency "energy" present on AC circuits, which are the frequencies most detrimental to human health.

The Stetzer meter is available at tinyurl.com/ExposedStetzer.

Advanced Meters

I use some advanced meters for special problems that occasionally arise. They are more expensive than the previously mentioned meters. You do not need them, unless you want to pursue becoming a Certified Electromagnetic Radiation Specialist.

Sources for advanced products are:

- ➢ Safe Living Technologies at slt.co. For 5% off, use coupon code safe7 at checkout.
- ➢ Less EMF at tinyurl.com/ExposedLessEMF.

Actions for Today:

- ✓ Consider investing in one or more meters.
- ✓ Know that you can do this, and that there are many resources to help you.

Need or want solutions right now?

Go to Chapters 7, 8 and 9 (more than 30 pages of solutions) and Appendix I for your Comprehensive Home Safety Audit.

Chapter 12

Safely Home
How Do We Know What Is Safe?

To identify safe levels for sleep areas, I use the Building Biology Guidelines (SBM 2015). Sleep areas are the most critical areas to control. For safety ranges for sleep areas, see the guidelines on page 199.

How are the guidelines determined?

These standards are based on the experience and knowledge of the Building Biology community, and the standards focus on achievability. In addition, scientific studies and other recommendations are consulted. With its professional approach, Building Biology testing methods help identify, minimize, and avoid environmental risk factors within an individual's framework of possibility.

Have the numbers changed over time?

Yes. With the mounting evidence of EMF harm, our standards have gotten stricter.

Have industry and governmental guidelines adjusted with the scientific evidence?

Internationally, some have changed. But the U.S. has not budged. The U.S. is living in the past on this—1996.

How do these safety standards compare with industry or governmental regulations?

Building Biology's acceptable levels of radiation are much, much lower. By a lot. By "lower" I mean that acceptable exposure levels have dropped and the standards are stricter. The "Concern" levels have been lowered because Building Biology health and safety standards are higher. There are several sources that provide interesting (and disturbing) comparisons of standards, country by country.

Check out:

- Safe Living Technologies: tinyurl.com/ExposedSafeLevels. Click on the International EMF Exposure Guidelines.
- General Public Exposure Standards or Guidelines for Several Countries or Agencies: tinyurl.com/ExposedPublicExposure.
- Compilation of EMF limits and standards worldwide: emfs.info/limits/world/.

If you take the time to look at all of the comparisons you may find some of the charts and numbers are a bit technical. But it doesn't take a degree in math or physics to see the difference. It should give you cause for a high level of concern about the "safety standards" listed for the U.S. You can see for yourself; in some categories, the safety standards in the U.S. are a thousand times higher than what we recommend and what has been adopted by other countries.

What do the recommended meters measure?

- The Safe and Sound Classic and Acousticom 2 measure Wireless/WiFi/Bluetooth/RF/ Microwave radiation. The Safe and Sound uses words to indicate levels of "Concern," and the Acousticom 2 measures in volts per meter (V/m). (They both measure radiation through the AIR from your wireless devices or cell towers.)
- Gigahertz ME3030B (on the E setting) measures electric radiation in volts per meter (V/m). (Measures electric radiation from your wires.)
- Gigahertz ME3030B (on the M setting) measures magnetic radiation in nanotesla (nT). (Measures magnetic radiation caused by the flow of electricity through your wires.)

- The Greenwave Meter measures dirty electricity in millivolts (mV). The Stetzer Meter measures dirty electricity in Graham–Stetzer Units (GS). (Both measure high-frequency voltage transients and harmonics; i.e., radiation that rides on your wires.)

Building Biology Guidelines (SBM 2015) for Sleep Areas

Type of Radiation	No Concern	Slight Concern	Severe Concern	Extreme Concern
Safe & Sound RF/WiFi/Wireless/Bluetooth	Slight-LED	Moderate-LED	High-LED	Extreme-LED
Acousticom 2 RF/WiFi/Wireless/Bluetooth	V/m <.01	.01 - .06	.06 - .61	> .61
Electric - V/m	<.03	.03 - 1.5	1.5 - 10	> 10
Magnetic - nT	<20	20 - 100	100 - 500	> 500

Different meters use different units of measurements. If you are not using the exact meters listed above, please go to this link to determine what the safe levels are: slt.co.

Please remember, if you are going to slt.co to purchase any items, use the coupon code safe7 to save 5%.

Greenwave Dirty Electricity Meter – mV

RECOMMENDED EMI (Electromagnetic Interference) LEVELS: Ideally, dirty electricity (EMI) levels should be below 25 millivolts (mV). Levels between 25 and 50 mV are marginal and should be reduced if possible. Levels above 50 mV are undesirable and steps should be taken to lower them.

A good rule of thumb is to reduce levels of dirty electricity to less than 50 mV. The lower you can get dirty electricity, the better.

I personally like to get under 30 mV in a sleep area with the use of dirty electricity filters.

Stetzer Dirty Electricity Meter – GS Units (Graham – Stetzer Units)

Less than 25 – Good
25 to 50 – Average
More than 50 – Undesirable

I like to get below 25 GS units in sleep areas and below 50 GS units in non-sleep areas.

Again, different meters use different units of measurements. If you are not using the ***exact meters*** listed above, please go to this link to determine the safe levels: slt.co.

Actions for Today:

- ✓ Use meters to verify that you are in the safer ranges.
- ✓ Make every effort to remediate radiation, especially in sleep areas.
- ✓ Before using dirty electricity filters, please review Three Bits of Caution on page 182.

Need or want solutions right now?

Go to Chapters 7, 8 and 9 (more than 30 pages of solutions) and Appendix I for your Comprehensive Home Safety Audit.

SECTION IV

Appendices & References

Appendix I

Comprehensive Home Safety Audit

We can't escape ALL EMR in our contemporary culture. But we can take a good chunk out of our daily exposure. I have assembled a list of devices that can produce radiation inside your home and outside your home.

There are two lists for radiation—through the AIR and from WIRES. They are arranged room by room.

It is the most comprehensive home audit I know of. It is exhaustive. I created it. And updated it based on my continuing education, my experience doing home, school, and business EMF inspections, and my annual visits to CES (Consumer Electronics Show).

This Home Safety Audit Report can be a little intimidating. It is a big, long list of items to look for, room by room. It is similar to what I use when I do an EMF inspection. What I use during a home, school, or business EMF inspection is a spreadsheet that includes "Concern" levels and an area for comments. I code the results so the client can quickly discern where the hot spots are, where moderate exposure exists, and where the green-clean areas are.

As you can see, it is very thorough. I go room by room and check for ALL types of EMR—through the AIR and from WIRES. Pay extra attention to your sleep area.

If you are new to this, I suggest just picking one room, such as the bedroom (or nursery, if you have a little one) and taking an audit of how many sources of EMR/EMF are present in that room. Take a few steps to reduce your exposure using the advice in Section II.

In most free-standing, single-family homes, I am able to reduce the EMR by more than 90 percent. YOU can do the same, with a little help from a Certified Electromagnetic Radiation Specialist.

Indentifying Potential Sources of Radiation Through the Air

Bedroom – WiFi/Wireless/Bluetooth/Smart Devices

Some of the below devices can have a WiFi, Wireless, Bluetooth or Smart component in them. Normally there is an interaction with a Smartphone.

☐ Air Filters – Smart
☐ Air Purifier
☐ Alarm Clock sound & vibration
☐ Anti-Snoring Device – Smart
☐ Bed Pad – Smart
☐ Bed Speakers
☐ Bedwetting Alarm
☐ Blu-ray DVD Player
☐ Cable Box
☐ Camera
☐ Ceiling Fan
☐ Ceiling Lamp with Speaker
☐ Ceiling Light Fixture
☐ Cell Phone
☐ Charger – Wireless
☐ Chargers
☐ Clock
☐ Control Buttons – Smart
☐ Cordless Phone
☐ CPAP Machines
☐ Digital Media Player
☐ Dimmer Switches
☐ Door Locks
☐ DVR
☐ Earbuds
☐ eBook Readers
☐ EKG Patch
☐ Essential Oil Diffuser
☐ Fan – Portable
☐ Fertility Tracker
☐ Fetal Monitor
☐ Fetus Camera
☐ Fetus Monitoring Band
☐ Fragrance Disseminator
☐ Gaming Systems
☐ Glasses – Smart
☐ HDTV Transmitter
☐ Headband Headset
☐ Head Phones – Wireless
☐ Heater – Portable

☐ Home Air Quality Monitor
☐ Home Audio
☐ Home Automation Item Tracker
☐ Home Devices – Smart
☐ Home Hub for all devices
☐ Home Sensing Carpet
☐ Intercom
☐ Internet Streaming Device
☐ Internet TV Device
☐ Internet Video Service
☐ iPad/Tablet/Kindle
☐ Lamps – Smart
☐ Laptop
☐ Light Bulb and Speaker
☐ Light Bulbs – Smart
☐ Light Switch
☐ Lighting Systems
☐ Mattress Cover – Smart
☐ Media Streamers
☐ Meditation Tracker
☐ Medical Monitoring
☐ Motion Detector
☐ Motorized Window Blinds
☐ MP3 Player
☐ Open or Close Door or Window Sensor
☐ Pillow for Snoring – Smart
☐ Plug Adaptor/Controller
☐ Power Strip – Smart
☐ Projector
☐ Remote Door Bell Chime
☐ Remote Thermostat Sensors
☐ Robot Vacuum
☐ Satellite Receiver
☐ Sauna
☐ Security Camera
☐ Security Lighting
☐ Security – Virtual Roommate
☐ Senior Home Health Monitoring
☐ Signal Booster/Extender
☐ Sleep Huggable Pillow
☐ Sleep monitoring System
☐ Sleeping Earphones
☐ Speakers – Smart
☐ Speakers – Wireless
☐ Thermostat – Smart
☐ TV
☐ TV Services
☐ Video Game Console
☐ Visual Enhancement Glasses
☐ Watch – Smart

Bedroom – Radiation from Wires – Electric Radiation, Magnetic Radiation & Dirty Electricity

☐ Plugged in Bluetooth Devices
☐ Plugged in WiFi Devices
☐ Plugged in Wireless Devices
☐ Plugged in Smart Devices

☐ Air Purifier
☐ Alarm Clock sound & vibration
☐ Bed Pad
☐ Bed Speakers
☐ Bedwetting Alarm
☐ Blu-ray DVD Player
☐ Cable Box
☐ Ceiling Fan
☐ Ceiling Lamp with Speaker
☐ Ceiling Light Fixture
☐ Charger - Wireless
☐ Chargers
☐ Clock
☐ Cordless Phone
☐ CPAP Machines
☐ Digital Media Player
☐ Dimmer Switches
☐ DVR
☐ Earbuds
☐ Electric Bed
☐ Electric Blanket
☐ Essential Oil Diffuser
☐ Extension Cords
☐ Fan – Portable
☐ Fragrance Disseminator
☐ Gaming Systems
☐ HDTV Transmitter
☐ Heater – Portable
☐ Heating Pad
☐ Home Air Quality Monitor
☐ Home Audio
☐ Home Automation Item Tracker
☐ Home Devices – Smart
☐ Home Hub for all devices
☐ Home Sensing Carpet
☐ Intercom
☐ Internet Streaming Device
☐ Internet TV Device
☐ Internet Video Service
☐ Lamps
☐ Light Bulb and Speaker
☐ Light Bulbs – Compact Fluorescent Lights (CFLs)
☐ Light Bulbs – Halogens – Small Base
☐ Light Bulbs – LEDs some
☐ Light Switch
☐ Lighting Systems
☐ Mattress Cover
☐ Media Streamers
☐ Meditation Tracker
☐ Medical Monitoring
☐ Motion Detector
☐ Motorized Window Blinds
☐ Plug Adaptor/Controller

- ☐ Power Strips
- ☐ Projector
- ☐ Remote Door Bell Chime
- ☐ Remote Thermostat Sensors
- ☐ Satellite Receiver
- ☐ Sauna
- ☐ Security – Virtual Roommate
- ☐ Security Camera
- ☐ Security Lighting
- ☐ Senior Home Health Monitoring
- ☐ Signal Booster/Extender
- ☐ Sleep Huggable Pillow
- ☐ Sleep monitoring System
- ☐ Sleeping Earphones
- ☐ Speakers
- ☐ Speakers – Smart
- ☐ Thermostat
- ☐ TV
- ☐ TV Services
- ☐ Video Game Console

Family Room/Living Room – WiFi/Wireless/ Bluetooth/Smart Devices

Some of the below devices can have a WiFi, Wireless, Bluetooth or Smart component in them. Normally there is an interaction with a Smartphone.

- ☐ Air Filters – Smart
- ☐ Air Purifier
- ☐ Blu-ray DVD Player
- ☐ Cable Box
- ☐ Ceiling Fan
- ☐ Ceiling Lamp with Speaker
- ☐ Ceiling Light Fixture
- ☐ Cell Phone
- ☐ Charger – Wireless
- ☐ Chargers
- ☐ Clock
- ☐ Cordless Phone
- ☐ Delivery Door – Smart
- ☐ Digital Media Player
- ☐ Dimmer Switches
- ☐ Door Locks
- ☐ DVR
- ☐ Earbuds
- ☐ eBook Readers
- ☐ Essential Oil Diffuser
- ☐ Fan – Portable
- ☐ Fragrance Disseminator
- ☐ Gaming Systems
- ☐ Glasses – Smart
- ☐ HDTV Transmitter
- ☐ Head Phones – Wireless
- ☐ Headband Headset
- ☐ Heater – Portable

☐ Home Air Quality Monitor
☐ Home Audio
☐ Home Automation Item Tracker
☐ Home Devices – Smart
☐ Home Sensing Carpet
☐ Humidifier – Portable
☐ Intercom
☐ Internet Streaming Device
☐ Internet TV Device
☐ Internet Video Service
☐ iPad/Tablet/Kindle
☐ Lamps – Smart
☐ Laptop
☐ Light Bulb and Speaker
☐ Light Bulbs – Smart
☐ Light Switch
☐ Lighting
☐ Lighting Systems
☐ Media Streamers
☐ Meditation Tracker
☐ Motion Detector
☐ Motorized Window Blinds
☐ MP3 Player
☐ Open or Closed Door or Window Sensor
☐ Plug Adaptor/Controller
☐ Projector
☐ Remote Door Bell Chime
☐ Remote Thermostat Sensors
☐ Robot Vacuum
☐ Satellite Receiver
☐ Sauna
☐ Security Camera
☐ Security Lighting
☐ Senior Home Health Monitoring
☐ Signal Booster/Extender
☐ Speakers – Smart
☐ Speakers – Wireless
☐ Standalone Streaming Services
☐ Thermostat – Smart
☐ TV
☐ TV Services
☐ Video Game Console
☐ Visual Enhancement Glasses
☐ Watch – Smart

Family Room/Living Room – Radiation from Wires – Electric Radiation, Magnetic Radiation & Dirty Electricity

☐ Plugged in Bluetooth Devices
☐ Plugged in WiFi Devices
☐ Plugged in Wireless Devices
☐ Plugged in Smart Devices

☐ Air Purifier
☐ Blu-ray DVD Player
☐ Cable Box
☐ Ceiling Fan
☐ Ceiling Lamp with Speaker
☐ Ceiling Light Fixture
☐ Ceiling Lights
☐ Charger – Wireless
☐ Chargers
☐ Clock
☐ Cordless Phone
☐ Digital Media Player
☐ Dimmer Switches
☐ DVR
☐ Essential Oil Diffuser
☐ Extension Cords
☐ Fan – Portable
☐ Fragrance Disseminator
☐ Gaming Systems
☐ HDTV Transmitter
☐ Heater – Portable
☐ Home Air Quality Monitor
☐ Home Audio
☐ Home Devices – Smart
☐ Home Hub for all devices
☐ Home Sensing Carpet
☐ Humidifier – Portable
☐ Internet Streaming Device
☐ Internet TV Device
☐ Internet Video Service
☐ Lamps
☐ Light Bulb and Speaker
☐ Light Bulbs – Compact Fluorescent Lights (CFLs)
☐ Light Bulbs – Halogens – Small Base
☐ Light Bulbs – LEDs some
☐ Light Switch
☐ Lighting
☐ Lighting Systems
☐ Media Streamers
☐ Meditation Tracker
☐ Motion Detector
☐ Motorized Window Blinds
☐ MP3 Player
☐ Plug Adaptor/Controller
☐ Power Strips
☐ Projector
☐ Remote Door Bell Chime
☐ Remote Thermostat Sensors
☐ Satellite Receiver
☐ Sauna
☐ Security – Virtual Roommate

☐ Security Camera
☐ Security Lighting
☐ Senior Home Health Monitoring
☐ Signal Booster/Extender
☐ Speakers
☐ Speakers – Smart
☐ Standalone Streaming Services
☐ TV
☐ TV Services
☐ Video Game Console

Home Office – WiFi/Wireless/Bluetooth/Smart Devices

Some of the below devices can have a WiFi, Wireless, Bluetooth or Smart component in them. Normally there is an interaction with a Smartphone.

☐ Air Filters – Smart
☐ Air Purifier
☐ Blu-ray DVD Player
☐ Cable Box
☐ Ceiling Fan
☐ Ceiling Lamp with Speaker
☐ Ceiling Light Fixture
☐ Cell Phone
☐ Charger – Wireless
☐ Chargers
☐ Clock
☐ Cloud Reusable Notebook
☐ Cordless Phone
☐ Digital Media Player
☐ Digitizer Pen
☐ Dimmer Switches
☐ Door Locks
☐ DVR
☐ Earbuds
☐ Ear Piece
☐ eBook Readers
☐ Essential Oil Diffuser
☐ Fan – Portable
☐ Fax Machine
☐ Fitness Chair
☐ Fragrance Disseminator
☐ Gaming Systems
☐ Glasses – Smart
☐ HDTV Transmitter
☐ Head Phones
☐ Headband Headset
☐ Headset
☐ Heater – Portable
☐ Home Air Quality Monitor
☐ Home Audio
☐ Home Automation Item Tracker
☐ Home Devices – Smart
☐ Home Hub for all devices
☐ Home Sensing Carpet
☐ Humidifier – Portable
☐ Intercom
☐ Internet Streaming Device
☐ Internet TV Device

☐ Internet Video Service
☐ iPad/Tablet/Kindle
☐ Keyboard - Wireless
☐ Label Maker
☐ Lamps – Smart
☐ Laptop
☐ Light Bulb and Speaker
☐ Light Bulbs – Smart
☐ Light Switch
☐ Lighting Systems
☐ Media Streamers
☐ Meditation Tracker
☐ Modem
☐ Motion Detector
☐ Motorized Window Blinds
☐ Mouse – Wireless
☐ MP3 Player
☐ Neckloops
☐ Open or Close Door or Window Sensor
☐ PC Tower
☐ Plug Adaptor/Controller
☐ Power Strip – Smart
☐ Printer
☐ Printer – 3D
☐ Projector
☐ Remote Door Bell Chime
☐ Remote Thermostat
Sensors
☐ Robot Vacuum
☐ Router
☐ Satellite Receiver
☐ Sauna
☐ Security – Virtual Roommate
☐ Security Camera
☐ Security Lighting
☐ Senior Home Health Monitoring
☐ Signal Booster/Extender
☐ Speakers – Wireless
☐ Speakers – Smart
☐ Standalone Streaming Services
☐ Telephone Headset - Wireless
☐ Thermostat – Smart
☐ TV
☐ TV Services
☐ Video Game Console
☐ Visual Enhancement Glasses
☐ Watch – Smart
☐ Wearable Posture Trainer
☐ White Board

Home Office – Radiation from Wires – Electric Radiation, Magnetic Radiation & Dirty Electricity

☐ Plugged in Bluetooth Devices
☐ Plugged in WiFi Devices
☐ Plugged in Wireless Devices
☐ Plugged in Smart Devices

☐ Air Purifier
☐ Blu-ray DVD Player
☐ Cable Box
☐ Ceiling Fan
☐ Ceiling Lamp with Speaker
☐ Ceiling Light Fixture
☐ Ceiling Lights
☐ Charger - Wireless
☐ Chargers
☐ Clock
☐ Cordless Phone
☐ Digital Media Player
☐ Dimmer Switches
☐ DVR
☐ Essential Oil Diffuser
☐ Extension Cords
☐ Fan – Portable
☐ Fax Machine
☐ Fitness Chair - Electronic
☐ Fragrance Disseminator
☐ Gaming Systems
☐ HDTV Transmitter
☐ Heater – Portable
☐ Home Air Quality Monitor
☐ Home Audio
☐ Home Devices – Smart
☐ Home Hub for all devices
☐ Home Sensing Carpet
☐ Humidifier – Portable
☐ Internet Streaming Device
☐ Internet TV Device
☐ Internet Video Service
☐ Label Maker
☐ Lamps
☐ Laptop
☐ Light Bulb and Speaker
☐ Light Bulbs – Compact Fluorescent Lights (CFLs)
☐ Light Bulbs – Halogens – Small Base
☐ Light Bulbs – LEDs some
☐ Light Switch
☐ Lighting Systems
☐ Media Streamers
☐ Modem
☐ Motorized Window Blinds
☐ PC Tower
☐ Plug Adaptor/Controller
☐ Power Strips
☐ Printer
☐ Printer – 3D
☐ Projector
☐ Remote Door Bell Chime
☐ Remote Thermostat Sensors
☐ Router
☐ Satellite Receiver

☐ Sauna
☐ Security – Virtual Roommate
☐ Security Camera
☐ Security Lighting
☐ Senior Home Health Monitoring
☐ Signal Booster/Extender
☐ Speakers
☐ Speakers – Smart
☐ Speakers – Wireless
☐ Standalone Streaming Services
☐ Telephone Headset - Wireless
☐ TV
☐ TV Services
☐ Video Game Console
☐ White Board – Electronic

Utility Meters – Wireless

☐ Utility Meter, Electric
☐ Utility Meter, Gas
☐ Utility Meter, Water

Utility Meters – Radiation from Wires and Pipes – Electric Radiation, Magnetic Radiation & Dirty Electricity

☐ Utility Meter, Electric
☐ Utility Meter, Gas
☐ Utility Meter, Water

Nursery – WiFi/Wireless/Bluetooth/Smart Devices

Some of the below devices can have a WiFi, Wireless, Bluetooth or Smart component in them. Normally there is an interaction with a Smartphone.

☐ Air Filters – Smart
☐ Air Purifier
☐ Alarm Clock sound & vibration
☐ Baby Bottle – Smart
☐ Baby Headset
☐ Baby Heart Rate and Oxygen Monitor
☐ Baby Monitor
☐ Baby Monitor Wrist Band
☐ Baby Projector
☐ Baby Robot
☐ Baby Rocker
☐ Baby Table Lamp – Smart
☐ Baby Temperature and Humidity Device
☐ Baby Vibrating Bed Mat
☐ Baby Wearables
☐ Bassinet or Crib
☐ Bath Water Temperature
☐ Bed
☐ Bed Pad – Smart
☐ Bed Speakers
☐ Bedwetting Alarm
☐ Bib – Smart
☐ Blanket – Kick-off alert
☐ Blu-ray DVD Player
☐ Breast Pump
☐ Cable Box
☐ Ceiling Fan
☐ Ceiling Lamp with Speaker
☐ Ceiling Light Fixture
☐ Cell Phone
☐ Charger – Wireless
☐ Chargers
☐ Child Car Seat
☐ Clock
☐ Cordless Phone
☐ Dancing Robot
☐ Diaper – Smart
☐ Digital Media Player
☐ Dimmer Switches
☐ Door Locks
☐ DVR
☐ eBook Readers
☐ EKG Patch
☐ Essential Oil Diffuser
☐ Fan – Portable
☐ Fertility Tracker
☐ Fetal Monitor
☐ Fetus Camera
☐ Fetus Monitoring Band
☐ Fragrance Disseminator
☐ Glasses – Smart
☐ HDTV Transmitter
☐ Heater – Portable
☐ Home Air Quality Monitor
☐ Home Audio
☐ Home Automation Item Tracker

☐ Home Devices – Smart
☐ Home Hub for all devices
☐ Home Sensing Carpet
☐ Humidifier – Portable
☐ Intercom
☐ Internet Streaming Device
☐ Internet TV Device
☐ Internet Video Service
☐ iPad/Tablet/Kindle
☐ Lamps – Smart
☐ Laptop
☐ Light Bulb and Speaker
☐ Light Bulbs – Smart
☐ Light Switch
☐ Lighting Systems
☐ Mattress Cover – Smart
☐ Media Streamers
☐ Medical monitoring
☐ Motion Detector
☐ Motorized Window Blinds
☐ MP3 Player
☐ Napper & Bouncer – Portable
☐ Nursery Environment Monitor
☐ Open or Close Door or Window Sensor
☐ Pacifier – Smart
☐ Plug Adaptor/Controller
☐ Power Strip – Smart
☐ Projector
☐ Remote Door Bell Chime
☐ Remote Thermostat Sensors
☐ Robot Vacuum
☐ Satellite Receiver
☐ Scale – Baby
☐ Security – Virtual Roommate
☐ Security Camera
☐ Security Lighting
☐ Signal Booster/Extender
☐ Sleep Huggable Pillow
☐ Sleep monitoring System
☐ Sleeping Earphones
☐ Sock – Baby Monitor
☐ Sound Systems
☐ Speakers – Wireless
☐ Speakers – Smart
☐ Spit-up Alert
☐ Standalone Streaming Services
☐ Stroller Speaker
☐ Temperature Monitoring Patch
☐ Thermostat – Smart
☐ TV
☐ TV Services
☐ Video Game Console
☐ Visual Enhancement Glasses
☐ Watch – Smart
☐ Wearable – Baby Monitor

Nursery – Radiation from Wires – Electric Radiation, Magnetic Radiation & Dirty Electricity

☐ Plugged in Bluetooth Devices
☐ Plugged in WiFi Devices
☐ Plugged in Wireless Devices
☐ Plugged in Smart Devices

☐ Air Purifier
☐ Alarm Clock sound & vibration
☐ Baby Monitor
☐ Baby Projector
☐ Baby Robot
☐ Baby Rocker
☐ Baby Table Lamp
☐ Baby Temperature and Humidity Device
☐ Baby Vibrating Bed Mat
☐ Bassinet or Crib
☐ Bed
☐ Bed Pad
☐ Bed Speakers
☐ Bedwetting Alarm
☐ Blu-ray DVD Player
☐ Cable Box
☐ Ceiling Fan
☐ Ceiling Lamp with Speaker
☐ Ceiling Light Fixture
☐ Ceiling Lights
☐ Charger – Wireless
☐ Chargers
☐ Clock
☐ Cordless Phone
☐ Dancing Robot
☐ Digital Media Player
☐ Dimmer Switches
☐ DVR
☐ Electric Bed
☐ Electric Blanket
☐ Essential Oil Diffuser
☐ Extension Cords
☐ Fan – Portable
☐ Fragrance Disseminator
☐ HDTV Transmitter
☐ Heater – Portable
☐ Heating Pad
☐ Home Air Quality Monitor
☐ Home Audio
☐ Home Devices – Smart
☐ Home Hub for all devices
☐ Home Sensing Carpet
☐ Humidifier – Portable
☐ Intercom
☐ Internet Streaming Device
☐ Internet TV Device
☐ Internet Video Service
☐ Lamps
☐ Light Bulb and Speaker
☐ Light Bulbs – Compact Fluorescent Lights (CFLs)
☐ Light Bulbs – Halogens – Small Base
☐ Light Bulbs – LEDs some
☐ Light Switch

☐ Lighting Systems
☐ Mattress Cover
☐ Media Streamers
☐ Medical monitoring
☐ Motion Detector
☐ Motorized Window Blinds
☐ Nursery Environment Monitor
☐ Pacifier – Smart
☐ Plug Adaptor/Controller
☐ Power Strips
☐ Projector
☐ Remote Door Bell Chime
☐ Remote Thermostat Sensors
☐ Satellite Receiver
☐ Scale – Baby
☐ Security – Virtual Roommate
☐ Security Camera
☐ Security Lighting
☐ Signal Booster/Extender
☐ Smart Home Hub for all devices
☐ Sound Systems
☐ Speakers
☐ Speakers – Smart
☐ Standalone Streaming Services
☐ TV
☐ TV Services
☐ Video Game Console

Personal/Wearable – WiFi/Wireless/Bluetooth/Smart Devices

Some of the below devices can have a WiFi, Wireless, Bluetooth or Smart component in them. Normally there is an interaction with a Smartphone.

☐ Activity Tracker
☐ Anti-Nausea Band
☐ Back Packs – Smart
☐ Belt – Smart
☐ Brain Activity Tracker
☐ Cell Phone
☐ Child Locator – Wearable
☐ Child's Bone Conduction Headphones
☐ Child's Smartphone Watch
☐ Child's Vital Signs Monitor
☐ Child's Wireless Microphone
☐ Cycling Glasses – Smart
☐ Diabetes Monitor
☐ Earbuds
☐ Ear Piece
☐ Earmuffs
☐ eBook Readers
☐ EEG Monitor
☐ EKG or ECG Monitor
☐ EKG Patch

☐ Fall/Safety Monitoring Lamp
☐ Fertility Monitor
☐ Fetus Camera
☐ Fetus Monitoring Band
☐ Fitness – Wearables
☐ Fitness Coach
☐ Fitness Trackers
☐ Gesture Control Device – Wearable
☐ Glasses – Smart
☐ Glasses – Camera
☐ Gloves for Gaming – Wireless
☐ Head Phones – Wireless
☐ Headband Headset
☐ Health – Wearables
☐ Hearing Aids
☐ Hearing Aid Ear Buds – Bluetooth
☐ Hearing Amplification – Long Range
☐ Hearing Implant inside ear
☐ Heart Rate Sensor
☐ Home Automation Item Tracker
☐ Horseback Rider Fall/Safety Monitor
☐ Intestinal Movement Tracker – Wireless
☐ iPad/Tablet/Kindle
☐ Laptop
☐ Luggage – Smart
☐ Massager – Smart
☐ Media Streamers
☐ Meditation Head Band – Smart
☐ Microphone – Wearable
☐ Migraine – Anti-stimulation
☐ Motion-Ring 3D space Recognition Sensor
☐ MP3 Player
☐ Neckloops
☐ Noise Cancelling Earbuds
☐ Pain Relief – Wearable
☐ Personal Environment Monitor
☐ Respiratory Monitor
☐ Ring – Smart
☐ Senior Home Health Monitoring
☐ Shoe Insole – Smart
☐ Shoes – Smart
☐ Speakers – Baseball Cap
☐ Speakers – Wearable
☐ Stroke Detection Device
☐ Sweat Sensing Monitor
☐ Ultrasound Scanner
☐ Underwear – Smart
☐ Virtual Reality/ Augmented Reality Glasses
☐ Visual Enhancement Glasses
☐ Watch – Smart
☐ Wearables – General

Personal/Wearable – Radiation from Wires – Electric Radiation, Magnetic Radiation & Dirty Electricity

☐ Plugged in Bluetooth Devices
☐ Plugged in WiFi Devices
☐ Plugged in Wireless Devices
☐ Plugged in Smart Devices

Fitness/Exercise/Exercise Room – WiFi/Wireless/ Bluetooth/Smart Devices

Some of the below devices can have a WiFi, Wireless, Bluetooth or Smart component in them. Normally there is an interaction with a Smartphone.

☐ Ab Wheel – Smart
☐ Aerobic Equipment
☐ Air Filters – Smart
☐ Air Purifier
☐ Basketballs – Smart
☐ Belly-Fat Sensor
☐ Bike Airbag Vest
☐ Bike Computer
☐ Bike Helmet – Smart
☐ Bike Stationary – Smart
☐ Bike Tracker
☐ Blu-ray DVD Player
☐ Boxing Punch Tracker
☐ Cable Box
☐ Calorie Intake Monitor
☐ Ceiling Fan
☐ Ceiling Lamp with Speaker
☐ Cell Phone
☐ Charger – Wireless
☐ Chargers
☐ Clock
☐ Cordless Phone
☐ Core Equipment – Smart
☐ Cycling Glasses – Smart
☐ Digital Media Player
☐ Dimmer Switches
☐ Door Locks
☐ Drone – Gesture Controlled – Wireless
☐ DVR
☐ Earbuds
☐ eBook Readers
☐ Exercise Equipment
☐ Exercise Hoop – Smart
☐ Fan – Portable
☐ Fitness Coach
☐ Fitness Skin Suit – Smart
☐ Fitness Trackers
☐ Fitness Wearables
☐ Fragrance Disseminator
☐ Gaming Systems
☐ Glasses – Smart
☐ Glove – Smart
☐ Golf Cart Follower – Smart

☐ HDTV Transmitter
☐ Head Phones – Wireless
☐ Headband Headset
☐ Health – Wearables
☐ Heater – Portable
☐ Home Air Quality Monitor
☐ Home Audio
☐ Home Automation Item Tracker
☐ Home Devices – Smart
☐ Home Hub for all devices
☐ Home Sensing Carpet
☐ Humidifier – Portable
☐ Intercom
☐ Internet Streaming Device
☐ Internet TV Device
☐ Internet Video Service
☐ iPad/Tablet/Kindle
☐ Jump Rope – Smart
☐ Laptop
☐ Light Bulb and Speaker
☐ Light Bulbs – Smart
☐ Light Switch
☐ Lighting Systems
☐ Media Streamers
☐ Motion Detector
☐ Motorized Window Blinds
☐ MP3 Player
☐ Neckloops
☐ Open or Closed Door or Window Sensor
☐ Pedometer – Bluetooth
☐ Plug Adaptor/Controller
☐ Power Strip – Smart
☐ Projector
☐ Pushup Stands – Smart
☐ Remote Thermostat Sensors
☐ Resistance Bands – Smart
☐ Respiratory Monitor
☐ Robot Vacuum
☐ Satellite Receiver
☐ Sauna
☐ Security – Virtual Roommate
☐ Security Camera
☐ Security Lighting
☐ Shoe Insole – Smart
☐ Shoes – Smart
☐ Signal Booster/Extender
☐ Snow Skiing Helmet – Smart
☐ Snow Skis – Smart
☐ Soccer Ball – Smart
☐ Speakers – Wireless
☐ Speakers – Smart
☐ Standalone Streaming Services
☐ Tennis Racket – Smart
☐ Thermostat – Smart
☐ Thyroid Gland Stimulation – Smart
☐ TV
☐ TV Services
☐ Underwear – Smart
☐ Video Game Console
☐ Virtual Reality Workout Googles
☐ Visual Enhancement Glasses

☐ Watch – Smart
☐ Water Bottle Speaker – Bluetooth
☐ Wearables
☐ Weight Lifting Equipment – Smart
☐ Yoga Exercise Mat – Smart

Fitness/Exercise Room – Radiation from Wires – Electric Radiation, Magnetic Radiation & Dirty Electricity

☐ Plugged in Bluetooth Devices
☐ Plugged in WiFi Devices
☐ Plugged in Wireless Devices
☐ Plugged in Smart Devices

☐ Air Purifier
☐ Bike Computer
☐ Blu-ray DVD Player
☐ Cable Box
☐ Ceiling Fan
☐ Ceiling Lamp with Speaker
☐ Charger - Wireless
☐ Chargers
☐ Clock
☐ Cordless Phone
☐ Dimmer Switches
☐ DVR
☐ Electric Aerobic Equipment
☐ Electric Core Equipment
☐ Electric Exercise Equipment
☐ Electric Weight Lifting Equipment
☐ Extension Cords
☐ Fan – Portable
☐ Fitness Trackers
☐ Fragrance Disseminator
☐ Gaming Systems
☐ HDTV Transmitter
☐ Heater – Portable
☐ Home Air Quality Monitor
☐ Home Audio
☐ Home Devices – Smart
☐ Home Hub for all devices
☐ Home Sensing Carpet
☐ Humidifier – Portable
☐ Intercom
☐ Internet Streaming Device
☐ Internet TV Device
☐ Internet Video Service
☐ Light Bulb and Speaker
☐ Light Bulbs – Compact Fluorescent Lights (CFLs)
☐ Light Bulbs – Halogens – Small Base
☐ Light Bulbs – LEDs some
☐ Light Switch
☐ Lighting Systems
☐ Media Streamers
☐ Motion Detector
☐ Motorized Window Blinds

☐ Plug Adaptor/Controller
☐ Power Strips
☐ Projector
☐ Remote Thermostat Sensors
☐ Satellite Receiver
☐ Sauna
☐ Security – Virtual Roommate
☐ Security Camera
☐ Security Lighting
☐ Signal Booster/Extender
☐ Smart Home Hub for all devices
☐ Speakers
☐ Speakers – Smart
☐ Standalone Streaming Services
☐ TV
☐ TV Services
☐ Video Game Console
☐ Yoga Exercise Mat

Pet – WiFi/Wireless/Bluetooth/Smart Devices

Some of the below devices can have a WiFi, Wireless, Bluetooth or Smart component in them. Normally there is an interaction with a Smartphone.

☐ Cat Exercise Machine Treadmill
☐ Dog Barking Control
☐ Fences
☐ Pet Activity Monitor
☐ Pet Bed
☐ Pet Camera
☐ Pet Door
☐ Pet Doorbell
☐ Pet Feeder
☐ Pet Food Bowl
☐ Pet Monitoring – Habits and Sleep
☐ Pet Monitoring – Location
☐ Pet Toys
☐ Pet Tracking Camera
☐ Pet Treat Dispenser - WiFi
☐ Pet Water Bowl
☐ Pet Wearable Video Camera
☐ Remote Reward Dog Trainer Treats
☐ Robot Pet Camera
☐ Sliding Glass Pet Door – Smart
☐ Smartphone – Dog Trainer

Pet – Radiation from Wires – Electric Radiation, Magnetic Radiation & Dirty Electricity

☐ Plugged in Bluetooth Devices
☐ Plugged in WiFi Devices
☐ Plugged in Wireless Devices
☐ Plugged in Smart Devices

Equine Devices

Some of the below devices can have a WiFi, Wireless, Bluetooth or Smart component in them. Normally there is an interaction with a Smartphone.

☐ Horse Saddle Movement Monitor
☐ Horseback Rider Fall/Safety Monitor
☐ Wireless Fences

Kitchen – WiFi/Wireless/Bluetooth/Smart Devices

Some of the below devices can have a WiFi, Wireless, Bluetooth or Smart component in them. Normally there is an interaction with a Smartphone.

☐ Air Filters – Smart
☐ Air Purifier
☐ Baking Scale
☐ Blender
☐ Blu-ray DVD Player
☐ Cable Box
☐ Ceiling Fan
☐ Ceiling Lamp with Speaker
☐ Ceiling Light Fixture
☐ Cell Phone
☐ Charger – Wireless
☐ Chargers
☐ Clock
☐ Coffee Maker
☐ Cooking System - Smart
☐ Cordless Phone
☐ Digital Media Player
☐ Dimmer Switches
☐ Dishwasher
☐ Door Locks
☐ DVR
☐ eBook Readers
☐ Essential Oil Diffuser
☐ Fan – Portable
☐ Fragrance Disseminator
☐ Freezer
☐ Frying Pan
☐ Glasses – Smart

- ☐ HDTV Transmitter
- ☐ Heater – Portable
- ☐ Home Air Quality Monitor
- ☐ Home Audio
- ☐ Home Automation Item Tracker
- ☐ Home Devices – Smart
- ☐ Home Hub for all devices
- ☐ Hot Water Kettle
- ☐ Humidifier – Portable
- ☐ Intercom
- ☐ Internet Streaming Device
- ☐ Internet TV Device
- ☐ Internet Video Service
- ☐ iPad/Tablet/Kindle
- ☐ Kitchen Scale
- ☐ Laptop
- ☐ Light Bulb and Speaker
- ☐ Light Bulbs – Smart
- ☐ Light Strips – Fluorescent
- ☐ Light Strips – LEDs
- ☐ Light Switch
- ☐ Lighting Systems
- ☐ Meat Thermometer – Smart
- ☐ Media Streamers
- ☐ Microwave Oven
- ☐ Motion Detector
- ☐ Motorized Window Blinds
- ☐ MP3 Player
- ☐ Open or Close Door or Window Sensor
- ☐ Plug Adaptor/Controller
- ☐ Power Strip – Smart
- ☐ Projector
- ☐ Refrigerator
- ☐ Refrigerator Camera
- ☐ Remote Door Bell Chime
- ☐ Remote Thermostat Sensors
- ☐ Robot Vacuum
- ☐ Satellite Receiver
- ☐ Security – Virtual Roommate
- ☐ Security Camera
- ☐ Security Lighting
- ☐ Senior Home Health Monitoring
- ☐ Signal Booster/Extender
- ☐ Slow Cooker
- ☐ Speakers – Wireless
- ☐ Speakers – Smart
- ☐ Standalone Streaming Services
- ☐ Stove
- ☐ Tea Kettle
- ☐ Temperature Probe
- ☐ Thermostat – Smart
- ☐ TV
- ☐ TV Services
- ☐ Video Game Console
- ☐ Visual Enhancement Glasses
- ☐ Watch – Smart
- ☐ Water Bottle – Smart
- ☐ Water Cooking – Smart
- ☐ Water Filtration System

Kitchen – Radiation from Wires – Electric Radiation, Magnetic Radiation & Dirty Electricity

- ☐ Plugged in Bluetooth Devices
- ☐ Plugged in WiFi Devices
- ☐ Plugged in Wireless Devices
- ☐ Plugged in Smart Devices
- ☐ Air Purifier
- ☐ Baking Scale
- ☐ Blender
- ☐ Blu-ray DVD Player
- ☐ Cable Box
- ☐ Ceiling Fan
- ☐ Ceiling Lamp with Speaker
- ☐ Ceiling Light Fixture
- ☐ Ceiling Lights
- ☐ Charger - Wireless
- ☐ Chargers
- ☐ Clock
- ☐ Coffee Maker
- ☐ Cooking System – Smart
- ☐ Cordless Phone
- ☐ Digital Media Player
- ☐ Dimmer Switches
- ☐ Dishwasher
- ☐ DVR
- ☐ Electric Frying Pan
- ☐ Electric Hot Water Kettle
- ☐ Electric Slow Cooker
- ☐ Essential Oil Diffuser
- ☐ Extension Cords
- ☐ Fan – Portable
- ☐ Fragrance Disseminator
- ☐ Freezer
- ☐ Frying Pan
- ☐ HDTV Transmitter
- ☐ Heater – Portable
- ☐ Home Air Quality Monitor
- ☐ Home Audio
- ☐ Home Devices – Smart
- ☐ Home Hub for all devices
- ☐ Humidifier
- ☐ Humidifier – Portable
- ☐ Intercom
- ☐ Internet Streaming Device
- ☐ Internet TV Device
- ☐ Internet Video Service
- ☐ Lamps
- ☐ Light Bulb and Speaker
- ☐ Light Bulbs – Compact Fluorescent Lights (CFLs)
- ☐ Light Bulbs – Halogens – Small Base
- ☐ Light Bulbs – LEDs some
- ☐ Light Strips – Fluorescent
- ☐ Light Strips – LEDs
- ☐ Light Switch
- ☐ Lighting Systems
- ☐ Media Streamers
- ☐ Microwave Oven
- ☐ Motion Dctector
- ☐ Motorized Window Blinds
- ☐ Plug Adaptor/Controller
- ☐ Power Strips
- ☐ Projector

- ☐ Refrigerator
- ☐ Refrigerator Camera
- ☐ Remote Door Bell Chime
- ☐ Remote Thermostat Sensors
- ☐ Satellite Receiver
- ☐ Security – Virtual Roommate
- ☐ Security Camera
- ☐ Security Lighting
- ☐ Senior Home Health Monitoring
- ☐ Signal Booster/Extender
- ☐ Speakers
- ☐ Speakers – Smart
- ☐ Standalone Streaming
- ☐ Stove
- ☐ Toaster Oven
- ☐ TV
- ☐ TV Services
- ☐ Video Game Console
- ☐ Visual Enhancement Glasses
- ☐ Water Cooking – Smart
- ☐ Water Filtration System, Electric

Car – WiFi/Wireless/Bluetooth/Smart Devices

Some of the below devices can have a WiFi, Wireless, Bluetooth or Smart component in them. Normally there is an interaction with a Smartphone.

- ☐ Advanced Intelligent Car Seat Monitoring
- ☐ Bluetooth Devices
- ☐ Car License Plate Frame
- ☐ Car Monitor – Drunk and Fatigue Driving
- ☐ Charger – Wireless
- ☐ Glasses – Smart
- ☐ MP3 Player
- ☐ Smart Devices
- ☐ Visor Speaker
- ☐ Watch – Smart
- ☐ WiFi Devices
- ☐ Wireless Devices

Car – Radiation from Wires – Electric Radiation, Magnetic Radiation & Dirty Electricity

- ☐ Anything you plug into a 2-prong or 3-prong adaptor in a car – 120 Volt Devices

Bathroom – WiFi/Wireless/Bluetooth/Smart Devices

Some of the below devices can have a WiFi, Wireless, Bluetooth or Smart component in them. Normally there is an interaction with a Smartphone.

☐ Air Filters – Smart
☐ Air Purifier
☐ Bathmat – Smart
☐ Bathroom Fan with Speaker
☐ Bathroom Humidity Sensor
☐ Bathroom Speakers
☐ Ceiling Fan
☐ Ceiling Lamp with Speaker
☐ Ceiling Light Fixture
☐ Cell Phone
☐ Charger – Wireless
☐ Chargers
☐ Clock
☐ Dimmer Switches
☐ Door Locks
☐ Earbuds
☐ eBook Readers
☐ Essential Oil Diffuser
☐ Fan – Portable
☐ Fragrance Disseminator
☐ Glasses – Smart
☐ HDTV Transmitter
☐ Head Phones – Wireless
☐ Heater – Portable
☐ Home Air Quality Monitor
☐ Home Audio
☐ Home Automation Item Tracker
☐ Home Devices – Smart
☐ Home Hub for all devices
☐ Humidifier – Portable
☐ Intercom
☐ iPad/Tablet/Kindle
☐ Light Bulb and Speaker
☐ Light Bulbs – Smart
☐ Light Switch
☐ Lighting Systems
☐ Media Streamers
☐ Mirror – Smart
☐ Motion Detector
☐ MP3 Player
☐ Open or Close Door or Window Sensor
☐ Plug Adaptor/Controller
☐ Power Strip – Smart
☐ Remote Door Bell Chime
☐ Remote Thermostat Sensors
☐ Robot Vacuum
☐ Scale – Adult
☐ Scale – Baby
☐ Sauna
☐ Security Camera
☐ Security Lighting
☐ Security – Virtual Roommate
☐ Senior Home Health Monitoring

☐ Signal Booster/Extender
☐ Speakers – Wireless
☐ Speakers – Smart
☐ Thermostat – Smart
☐ Toothbrush – Smart
☐ Visual Enhancement Glasses
☐ Watch – Smart

Bathroom – Radiation from Wires – Electric Radiation, Magnetic Radiation & Dirty Electricity

☐ Plugged in Bluetooth Devices
☐ Plugged in WiFi Devices
☐ Plugged in Wireless Devices
☐ Plugged in Smart Devices

☐ Air Purifier
☐ Bathroom Fan with Speaker
☐ Bathroom Humidity Sensor
☐ Bathroom Speakers
☐ Ceiling Fan
☐ Ceiling Lamp with Speaker
☐ Ceiling Light Fixture
☐ Charger – Wireless
☐ Chargers
☐ Clock
☐ Curling Iron
☐ Dimmer Switches
☐ Electric Shaver
☐ Electric Shaver Charger
☐ Electric Toothbrush Holder
☐ Essential Oil Diffuser
☐ Extension Cords
☐ Fan – Portable
☐ Fragrance Disseminator
☐ Hair Dryer
☐ HDTV Transmitter
☐ Heater – Portable
☐ Home Air Quality Monitor
☐ Home Audio
☐ Home Devices – Smart
☐ Home Hub for all devices
☐ Humidifier – Portable
☐ Intercom
☐ Light Bulb and Speaker
☐ Light Bulbs – Compact Fluorescent Lights (CFLs)
☐ Light Bulbs – Halogens – Small Base
☐ Light Bulbs – LEDs some
☐ Light Switch
☐ Lighted Vanity Mirror
☐ Lighting Systems
☐ Media Streamers
☐ Motion Detector
☐ Plug Adaptor/Controller
☐ Power Strip

- ☐ Remote Door Bell Chime
- ☐ Remote Thermostat Sensors
- ☐ Sauna
- ☐ Security – Virtual Roommate
- ☐ Security Camera
- ☐ Security Lighting
- ☐ Senior Home Health Monitoring
- ☐ Signal Booster/Extender
- ☐ Speakers
- ☐ Speakers – Smart Services
- ☐ TV
- ☐ TV Services
- ☐ Video Game Console
- ☐ Visual Enhancement Glasses

Outside/Patio – WiFi/Wireless/Bluetooth/Smart Devices

Some of the below devices can have a WiFi, Wireless, Bluetooth or Smart component in them. Normally there is an interaction with a Smartphone.

- ☐ Blu-ray DVD Player
- ☐ Cable Box
- ☐ Ceiling Fan
- ☐ Ceiling Lamp with Speaker
- ☐ Ceiling Light Fixture
- ☐ Cell Phone
- ☐ Charger – Wireless
- ☐ Chargers
- ☐ Clock
- ☐ Cordless Phone
- ☐ Delivery Door - Smart
- ☐ Digital Media Player
- ☐ Dimmer Switches
- ☐ Door Bell
- ☐ Door Locks
- ☐ DVR
- ☐ eBook Readers
- ☐ Essential Oil Diffuser
- ☐ Fan – Portable
- ☐ Flower Pot with Speakers
- ☐ Fragrance Disseminator
- ☐ Gaming Systems
- ☐ Garden Sensor
- ☐ Gas Leak Detector
- ☐ Glasses – Smart
- ☐ HDTV Transmitter
- ☐ Head Phones – Wireless
- ☐ Heater – Portable
- ☐ Home Audio
- ☐ Home Automation Item Tracker
- ☐ Home Devices – Smart
- ☐ Home Hub for all devices
- ☐ Humidifier – Portable
- ☐ Ice Cooler with Speakers
- ☐ Intelligent Lock Box
- ☐ Intercom
- ☐ Internet Streaming Device

☐ Internet TV Device
☐ Internet Video Service
☐ iPad/Tablet/Kindle
☐ Irrigation System
☐ Lamps – Smart
☐ Laptop
☐ Light Bulb and Speaker
☐ Light Bulbs – Smart
☐ Light Switch
☐ Lighting
☐ Lighting Systems
☐ Meat Thermometer – Smart
☐ Media Streamers
☐ Medical monitoring
☐ Meditation Tracker
☐ Microphone
☐ Motion Detector
☐ MP3 Player
☐ Open or Close Door or Window Sensor
☐ Outdoor Grill
☐ Outdoor Hub
☐ Outdoor Lights with Speakers
☐ Outdoor Lock
☐ Outdoor Motion Detectors
☐ Outdoor Smoker
☐ Patio Daybed
☐ Patio Heater
☐ Patio Heater with Speakers
☐ Plug Adaptor/Controller
☐ Power Strip – Smart
☐ Projector
☐ Propane Tank Level Monitor
☐ Remote Door Bell Chime
☐ Remote Thermostat Sensors
☐ Satellite Receiver
☐ Sauna
☐ Security Camera
☐ Security Lighting
☐ Senior Home Health Monitoring
☐ Signal Booster/Extender
☐ Speakers – Wireless
☐ Speakers – Smart
☐ Speakers in Spa
☐ Standalone Streaming Services
☐ Thermostat – Smart
☐ TV
☐ TV Services
☐ Umbrella Speakers

☐ Utility Meter, Electric
☐ Utility Meter, Gas
☐ Utility Meter, Water

☐ Video Game Console
☐ Visual Enhancement Glasses
☐ Watch – Smart
☐ Water Bottle – Smart
☐ Water Leak Detector
☐ Weather Station

Outside/Patio – Radiation from Wires – Electric Radiation, Magnetic Radiation & Dirty Electricity

☐ Plugged in Bluetooth Devices
☐ Plugged in WiFi Devices
☐ Plugged in Wireless Devices
☐ Plugged in Smart Devices

☐ Buried Power Lines
☐ Cable TV Line
☐ Overhead Power Lines
☐ Telephone Line
☐ Utility Meter, Electric
☐ Utility Meter, Gas
☐ Utility Meter, Water
☐ Water Line

☐ Blu-ray DVD Player
☐ Cable Box
☐ Cable TV Line
☐ Ceiling Fan
☐ Ceiling Fans
☐ Ceiling Lamp with Speaker
☐ Ceiling Light Fixture
☐ Charger – Wireless
☐ Chargers
☐ Clock – Electric
☐ Cordless Phone
☐ Digital Media Player
☐ Dimmer Switches
☐ DVR
☐ Electric Outdoor Grill/Smoker
☐ Electric Patio Daybed
☐ Electric Patio Heater
☐ Electric Patio Heater with Bluetooth Speakers
☐ Essential Oil Diffuser
☐ Extension Cords
☐ Fan – Portable
☐ Fragrance Disseminator
☐ Gaming Systems
☐ HDTV Transmitter
☐ Heater – Portable
☐ Home Audio
☐ Home Devices – Smart
☐ Home Hub for all devices
☐ Humidifier – Portable
☐ Ice Cooler with Speakers
☐ Intelligent Lock Box
☐ Intercom
☐ Internet Streaming Device
☐ Internet TV Device
☐ Internet Video Service
☐ Irrigation System
☐ Irrigation System Controller
☐ Lamps
☐ Light Bulb and Speaker
☐ Light Bulbs – Compact Fluorescent Lights (CFLs)
☐ Light Bulbs – Halogens – Small Base
☐ Light Bulbs – LEDs some
☐ Light Switch

☐ Lighting
☐ Lighting Systems
☐ Media Streamers
☐ Medical monitoring
☐ Meditation Tracker
☐ Microphone
☐ Motion Detector
☐ Outdoor Grill
☐ Outdoor Hub
☐ Outdoor Lights with Speakers
☐ Outdoor Motion Detectors
☐ Outdoor WiFi Hub
☐ Patio Daybed
☐ Patio Heater
☐ Patio Heater with Speakers
☐ Plug Adaptor/Controller
☐ Power Strip
☐ Projector
☐ Remote Door Bell Chime
☐ Remote Thermostat Sensors
☐ Satellite Receiver
☐ Sauna
☐ Security Camera
☐ Security Lighting
☐ Senior Home Health Monitoring
☐ Signal Booster/Extender
☐ Speakers
☐ Speakers – Smart
☐ Speakers in Spa
☐ Standalone Streaming Services
☐ Thermostat
☐ TV
☐ TV Services
☐ Video Game Console
☐ Water Leak Detector

Garage/Basement – WiFi/Wireless/Bluetooth/Smart Devices

Some of the below devices can have a WiFi, Wireless, Bluetooth or Smart component in them. Normally there is an interaction with a Smartphone.

- ☐ Driveway Alert – Smart
- ☐ Garage Door Opener
- ☐ Home Audio
- ☐ Home Devices – Smart
- ☐ Irrigation Clock
- ☐ Power Strip – Smart
- ☐ Sauna
- ☐ Tools – Smart
- ☐ Water Filtration System
- ☐ Water Leak Detector
- ☐ Water Softener
- ☐ Weather Station

Garage/Basement – Radiation from Wires – Electric Radiation, Magnetic Radiation & Dirty Electricity

- ☐ Plugged in Bluetooth Devices
- ☐ Plugged in WiFi Devices
- ☐ Plugged in Wireless Devices
- ☐ Plugged in Smart Devices

- ☐ Extension Cords
- ☐ Garage Door Opener
- ☐ Home Audio
- ☐ Home Devices – Smart
- ☐ Irrigation Clock
- ☐ Light Bulbs – Compact Fluorescent Lights (CFLs)
- ☐ Light Bulbs – Halogens – Small Base
- ☐ Light Bulbs – LEDs some
- ☐ Power Strip
- ☐ Sauna
- ☐ Water Filtration System
- ☐ Water Leak Detector
- ☐ Water Softener
- ☐ Weather Station

Laundry Room – WiFi/Wireless/Bluetooth/Smart Devices

Some of the below devices can have a WiFi, Wireless, Bluetooth or Smart component in them. Normally there is an interaction with a Smartphone.

- ☐ Air Filters – Smart
- ☐ Air Purifier
- ☐ Ceiling Fans
- ☐ Ceiling Lamp with Speaker
- ☐ Ceiling Light Fixture
- ☐ Cell Phone
- ☐ Charger – Wireless
- ☐ Chargers
- ☐ Clock
- ☐ Cordless Phone
- ☐ Dimmer Switches
- ☐ Door Locks
- ☐ Dryer
- ☐ Essential Oil Diffuser
- ☐ Fan – Portable
- ☐ Fragrance Disseminator
- ☐ Glasses – Smart
- ☐ HDTV Transmitter
- ☐ Heater – Portable
- ☐ Home Air Quality Monitor
- ☐ Home Audio
- ☐ Home Devices – Smart
- ☐ Home Hub for all devices
- ☐ Humidifier – Portable
- ☐ Intercom
- ☐ Lamps
- ☐ Light Bulb and Speaker
- ☐ Light Bulbs – Smart
- ☐ Light Switch
- ☐ Lighting
- ☐ Lighting Systems
- ☐ Motion Detector
- ☐ Open or Closed Door or Window Sensor
- ☐ Plug Adaptor/Controller
- ☐ Remote Door Bell Chime
- ☐ Remote Thermostat Sensors
- ☐ Robot Vacuum
- ☐ Security Camera
- ☐ Security Lighting
- ☐ Security – Virtual Roommate
- ☐ Signal Booster/Extender
- ☐ Speakers – Wireless
- ☐ Speakers – Smart
- ☐ Thermostat – Smart
- ☐ TV
- ☐ Washer
- ☐ Watch – Smart

Laundry Room – Radiation from Wires – Electric Radiation, Magnetic Radiation & Dirty Electricity

☐ Plugged in Bluetooth Devices
☐ Plugged in WiFi Devices
☐ Plugged in Wireless Devices
☐ Plugged in Smart Devices

☐ Air Purifier
☐ Ceiling Fans
☐ Ceiling Lamp with Speaker
☐ Ceiling Light Fixture
☐ Charger – Wireless
☐ Chargers
☐ Clock
☐ Cordless Phone
☐ Dimmer Switches
☐ Dryer
☐ Essential Oil Diffuser
☐ Extension Cords
☐ Fan – Portable
☐ Fragrance Disseminator
☐ HDTV Transmitter
☐ Heater – Portable
☐ Home Air Quality Monitor
☐ Home Audio
☐ Home Devices – Smart
☐ Home Hub for all devices
☐ Humidifier – Portable
☐ Intercom
☐ Lamps
☐ Light Bulb and Speaker
☐ Light Bulbs – Compact Fluorescent Lights (CFLs)
☐ Light Bulbs – Halogens – Small Base
☐ Light Bulbs – LEDs some
☐ Light Switch
☐ Lighting
☐ Lighting Systems
☐ Motion Detector
☐ Plug Adaptor/Controller
☐ Power Strip
☐ Remote Door Bell Chime
☐ Remote Thermostat Sensors
☐ Security – Virtual Roommate
☐ Security Camera
☐ Security Lighting
☐ Signal Booster/Extender
☐ Speakers
☐ Speakers – Smart
☐ TV
☐ Washer

Appendix II

More Questions? Resources for Advanced Reading

Books Documenting the Suppression and Cover-up of the Truth

Cell Phones: Invisible Hazards in the Wireless Age. George Carlo and Martin Schram. New York: Avalon, 2001.

Cell Phones and The Dark Deception: Find Out What You're Not Being Told . . . And Why. Carleigh Cooper. Grandville, MI: Premier Advantage Publishing, 2009.

Corporate Ties That Bind: An Examination of Corporate Manipulation and Vested Interest in Public Health. edited by Martin J. Walker, New York, NY: Skyhorse Publishing, Inc., March 28, 2017.

Currents of Death: Power Lines, Computer Terminals, and the Attempt to Cover Up Their Threats to Your Health. Paul Brodeur. New York, NY: Simon & Schuster; First Edition, 1989. Also available in paperback.

Disconnect, The Truth About Cell Phone Radiation. Dr. Devra Davis, New York, NY: Environmental Health Trust, 2013.

Going Somewhere, The Truth About a Life in Science. Andrew Marino, PhD, JD. Belcher, LA: Cassandra Publishing, 2010.

Truth About Cell Phone Radiation, What the Industry is Doing to Hide It, and How to Protect your Family, The. Dr. Devra Davis. New York, NY: Dutton, 2010.

Books About the Hazards of and Solutions to EMR/EMF

Cell Phones: Invisible Hazards in the Wireless Age: An Insider's Alarming Discoveries about Cancer and Genetic Damage. George Carlo and Martin Schram. Basic Books, 2002. First edition published by Avalon, 2001.

Cross Currents: The Perils of Electropollution, the Promise of Electromedicine. Robert O. Becker. Los Angeles, CA; Jeremy P. Tarcher, reprinted edition, 2004. First edition published by Penguin, 1990.

Disconnect, The Truth About Cell Phone Radiation. Dr. Devra Davis, New York, NY: Environmental Health Trust, 2013.

Electronic Silent Spring, An. Katie Singer. Great Barrington, MA: Portal Books, 2014.

Electromagnetic Fields: A Consumer's Guide to the Issues and How to Protect Ourselves, 2nd edition. Levitt, B. Blake. New York: Harcourt Brace, 2007.

EMF Freedom, Solutions for the 21st Century Pollution, 3rd Edition. Elizabeth Plourde, PhD, and Marcus Plourde, PhD. Irvine, CA: New Voice Publications, 2016.

Invisible Disease: The Dangers of Environmental Illnesses Caused by Electromagnetic Fields and Chemical Emissions, The. Gunni Nordstrom, O Books, John Hunt, 2004.

Non-Tinfoil Guide to EMFs: How to Fix Our Stupid Use of Technology, The. Nicolas Pineault. N&G Média, Inc., 2017.

Overpowered: The Dangers of Electromagnetic Radiation (EMF) and What You Can Do About It. Martin Blank. Seven Stories Press, Reprint edition, 2015.

Public Health SOS: The Shadow Side of the Wireless Revolution—110 Questions on Electromagnetic Pollution from a Forum at the Commonwealth Club of California. Magda Havas, PhD. Boulder, CO: Wide Angle Health, 2009.

Radiation Nation: Fallout of Modern Technology—Your Complete Guide to EMF Protection & Safety: The Proven Health Risks of Electromagnetic Radiation (EMF) & What to Do Protect

Yourself & Family. Daniel T. DeBaun and Ryan DeBaun. Icaro Publishing, 2017.

Wireless Radiation Rescue – 2012 (Revised & Updated Edition) How To Use Cell Phones More Safely and Other Safer-Tech Solutions. Kerry Crofton. Global Wellbeing Books, Third Edition, 2011.

Zapped: Why Your Cell Phone Shouldn't Be Your Alarm Clock and 1,268 Ways to Outsmart the Hazards of Electronic Pollution. Ann Louise Gittleman. New York, NY: McGraw-Hill Education, 2010.

History of Electricity and How We Got to Where We Are

Body Electric. Electromagnetism and the Foundation of Life, The (with Gary Selden). New York: NY: William Morrow & Co., Inc.; 1st edition, January 1, 1985. Also available in paperback and Kindle editions.

Dirty Electricity—Electrification and the Diseases of Civilization. Dr. Samuel Milham. iUniverse.com, 2010; 2nd Edition, 2012.

Invisible Rainbow, A History of Electricity and Life, The. Arthur Firstenberg. Santa Fe, NM: AGB Press, 2017.

Books and Articles That Deal With the Social, Emotional and Cultural Impact of Technology

Digital Cocaine: A Journey Toward iBalance [eBook]. Brad Huddleston. Christian Art Publishers, 2016.

Glow Kids: How Screen Addiction Is Hijacking Our Kids—and How to Break the Trance. Kardaras, Nicholas. Kindle Edition, New York, NY: St, Martin's Press, 2016.

Owned: Property, Privacy and the New Digital Serfdom. Joshua A. T. Fairfield. New York, NY: Cambridge University Press, 2017.

Screen Time Syndrome: Brain Images Explain Why Kids Are Moody, Impulsive & Can't Pay Attention. Jacqueline. October 9, 2017: deeprootsathome.com/screen-time-childs-brain.

Appendix III

Websites & Other Resources to Keep You Up-to-Date on the Inside Story

StopDirtyElectricity.com. Bill Cadwallader, MBA, EMRS—that's me!

Antenna Search: antennasearch.com. Type your address in the search box and see how many cell towers are in your neighborhood within a four-mile radius.

BioInitiative: bioinitiative.org. A report by 29 independent scientists and health experts (MDs and PhDs) from around the world gathering research about possible risks from wireless technologies and electromagnetic fields. Includes more than 3800 studies conducted worldwide. Editors: Cindy Sage and David Carpenter.

California Brain Tumor Association Facebook page: facebook.com/CALIBTA/. Consistent, up-to-date posts.

Canadians for Safe Technology: c4st.org. Good information on Electrosensitivity, as well as other related topics.

Cellular Phone Task Force: cellphonetaskforce.org. Features Education, Advocacy, Support. Arthur Firstenberg is the founder of this group and serves on its board of directors.

Central Brain Tumor Registry of the United States: cbtrus.org. Do you want to research the research? This is scientific, peer-reviewed research available for you to read for yourself.

Electrical Pollution: electricalpollution.com. Contains news, research, and tips on how you can take action on legislation and get involved in safety advocacy.

ElectricSense: electricsense.com. Lloyd Burrell offers many valuable podcasts. He has extensive knowledge on electromagnetic hypersensitivity (EHS).

Electromagnetic Health: electromagnetichealth.org. This website offers useful videos and audios from experts. Also has up-to-date news.

Electromagnetic Radiation Safety: saferemr.com. Dr. Joel Moskowitz, director, is an outspoken safety advocate. He is in the forefront of freedom of information and right to know regarding EMF safety issues.

Electronic Silent Spring: electronicsilentspring.com/may-2017-newsletter/. Published by Katie Singer, author of the book *An Electronic Silent Spring*, (2014).

EMF Facts Consultancy: emfacts.com. Independent information on the possible health and safety issues arising from human exposure to electromagnetic energy.

EMF-Portal: emf-portal.org/en. Summarizes systematically scientific research data on the effects of electromagnetic fields (EMF). The core of the EMF-Portal is an extensive literature database with an inventory of some 26,000 publications and 6,000 summaries of individual scientific studies on the effects of electromagnetic fields.

EMF Warriors YouTube Channel: youtube.com/channel/UCS_3NNeffxGd8uWO DCdKI9w. Has tons of fabulous interviews, including Andrew Marino.

Environmental Health Trust: ehtrust.org. Dr. Devra Davis, founder and president. This website not only contains valuable and reliable information, but also ideas on how you can take local action in your schools and community. It even has a resource for kids.

Firstenberg, Arthur: The Largest Biological Experiment Ever: proliberty.com/observer/20070307.htm. Arthur Firstenberg is an outspoken activist and expert. He wrote the book *The Invisible Rainbow, A History of Electricity and Life*, listed in Appendix II.

Generation Zapped: generationzapped.com/team/. Features the documentary film directed by Sabine El Gemayel, "Generation Zapped." This features an outstanding team of experts.

Greenwave International: greenwavefilters.com. Greenwave offers products and tips for reducing dirty electricity and other electropollution in homes, schools, businesses, and other settings. Our mission: Creating healthier spaces for living, learning, work, and more. For 5% percent off Greenwave products, use coupon code safe7 at checkout.

GUARDS (Global Union Against Radiation Deployment from Space: stopglobalWiFi.org. GUARDS is an international coalition against global WiFi from space, a complex technology of radiation and toxic chemicals endangering all life on Earth. Studies show radiation from wireless technology harms the environment—both flora and fauna are affected.

Downloads:

- moef.nic.in/downloads/public-information/final_mobile_towers_report.pdf
- biolmedonline.com/Articles/Vol4_4_2012/Vol4_4_202-216_BM-8.pdf

Havas, Magda, PhD: magdahavas.com. An expert. She speaks with authority on just about all topics related to EMR.

Healthy Homes Environmental: healthyhomesenvironmental.com. Farren Lander (British Columbia, Canada) works to reduce electropollution to healthy and acceptable levels, creating a safe haven for you and your family.

International EMF Alliance: iemfa.org/news/. This website pulls information from all over the world.

Kim Komando Show: komando.com/the-show. Kim has outstanding interviews of EMF experts on a variety of subjects.

Less EMF—The EMF Safety Shop: tinyurl.com/ExposedLessEMF. Online warehouse for gaussmeters, EMF meters and electromagnetic field shielding.

Manhattan Neighbors for Safer Telecommunications: manhattanneighbors.org/parents-schools/. Contains useful advice for parents and schools.

Mercola—Take Control of Your Health: emf.mercola.com. Dr. Mercola has some good videos available and provides excellent commentary on this topic.

Microwave News: microwavenews.com . Microwave News reports on the potential health and environmental impacts of EMFs. It is a consistently reliable source of news on this topic.

National Toxicology Program, U.S. Department of Health and Human Services

- "Telephone Press Conference: NTP Draft Conclusions for Radiofrequency Radiation Studies in Rats and Mice," February 2, 2018, niehs.nih.gov/news/newsroom/releases/2018/february 2/radiofrequency_508.pdf.
- "Draft Reports, Public Comments, and Related Information: TR Peer Review Panel," ntp.niehs.nih.gov/about/org/sep/trpanel/meetings/doc s/2018/march/index.html.

"National Toxicology Program (NTP) Cell Phone Radiation 2-Year Study—Evaluation of Carcinogenicity of Cell Phone Radiation: NTP Draft Technical Reports (TR 595, TR 596) vs. Expert Panel Vote," Joel M. Moskowitz, PhD, School of Public Health, UC Berkeley, March 28, 2018, emfsa.co.za/wp-content/uploads/2018/03/180328_ summary-of-NTP-expert-panel-recommendations.pdf.

One Radio Network: Live talk radio from the Texas Hill Country, oneradionetwork.com. I highly recommend his interviews with EMF experts.

OpenSecrets.org—Center for Responsive Politics: opensecrets.org. Valuable website allowing access to information about lobbying and campaign contributions.

Powerwatch: powerwatch.org.uk. Powerwatch gathers information from around the world about EMF in order to help the lay person understand this complex issue.

"Report on National Toxicology Program's Cell Phone Study," Arthur Firstenberg, April 12, 2018. cellphonetaskforce.org/ wp-content/uploads/2018/04/NTP-analysis.pdf.

Safe Living Technologies: slt.co. EMF/RF Measurement and Mitigation Specialists. For 5% off, use coupon code safe7 at checkout.

Scientists for Wired Technology: scientists4wiredtech.com. Advocacy based on scientists' research into the hazards of pulsed, data-modulated, Radiofrequency Microwave Radiation

Sensory Perspective – Detect + Protect in the Wireless World: detect-protect.com/k/. Features an excellent video, "She Looks Safe." You might have to click the scrolling banner to find it. Turn up the volume and be prepared to be alarmed.

StopDirtyElectricity.com. Bill Cadwallader, MBA, EMRS—that's me!

Take Back Your Power: takebackyourpower.net. This is a great organization exposing the truth about smart meters. Associated with Josh del Sol's documentary, "Take Back Your Power." Lots of ideas on how you can take action. Includes interesting videos.

Tobacco timelines:

- Tobacco Timeline at Sutori, sutori.com\\story\\tobacco-timeline-6bc8.
- "From Marlboro Man to Smoking Ban: A Timeline of Tobacco in America" by David Lawler, The Telegraph, 2014, telegraph.co.uk/news/worldnews/northamerica/usa/11230175/From-Marlboro-Man-to-smoking-ban-a-timeline-of-tobacco-in-America.html.
- Notabacco Center, Tobacco history headlines, notabaco.tripod.com/notabacocenter/id4.html.
- Tobacco Timeline: The Twentieth Century 1900-1949—The Rise of the Cigarette, author: Gene Borio, scribd.com/document/328812194/Tobacco-Timeline.

Certified Electromagnetic Radiation Specialists

Cadwallader, Bill. StopDirtyElectricity.com—that's me! – Nevada, Arizona, Utah, Southern California.

Burmaster, Spark. sparkburmaster.com – Wisconsin.
Doyon, Paul. ElectromagneticSafePlanet.com – California.
Gust, Larry. Gustenviro.com – California.
Menkes, Liz. EMFHealthy.com – California.
Metzinger, Rob. slt.co – Ontario, Canada.
Miller, Oram. CreateHealthyHomes.com – California.
Sagula, Lee. HealthyHomesConsulting.com – Pennsylvania.
Schultz, Diana. GreenAndHealthyHomes.net – Florida.
Windheim, Eric. WindheimEMFSolutions.com – California.

For more Certified Electromagnetic Radiation Specialists, go to hbelc.org/find-an-expert.

Appendix IV

Recommendations for limiting wireless technology pending further study and the development of safeguards against a potential threat to public health.

- Opinion from Olle Johansson: "Kick out politicians who give students hazardous e-readers"
- Scientists Warn of Potential Serious Health Impacts of 5G to Radiofrequency Energy from Cell Phones

Opinion from Olle Johansson

KI-researcher: kick out politicians who give students hazardous e-readers with unproven educational value

Sweden, 2014

Thanks to the so-called PISA* (OECD's Programme for International Student Assessment) survey, in Sweden we now know: student scores in maths, reading comprehension and natural sciences are plummeting. The results are prompting rage in Swedish schools. Something is wrong.

The government response is to force all students to go through another school year. In addition, a series of panic measures has been initiated by the authorities. But do not expect schools to be given peace and quiet, so that they may be able to figure out how to get things to work while dismantling those gadgets and administrative 'reins' that do not.

For years schools have undergone a multitude of changes and been given new assignments, including being forced to monitor more grade control data and using new and more administration. Some changes are good, some bad. Changes include an enormous amount of computerized teaching where students via their apps, mobile phones and tablets are supposed to gain new knowledge. Pedagogy innovators have deleted textbooks and pencils, blackboards and pointers, and instead replaced them with new wireless e-readers and cell phones. Academics, such as myself, have many times – usually completely unheard – raised a warning finger to the educational establishment.

Today it is very difficult to be a teacher and take responsibility for teaching in the classroom where students' cell phones are constantly ringing, text messages are being sent back and forth, and surfing the entire time online or playing games through iPhones and iPads. All this when students really should be working on their school assignments.

In Sweden, there have been several cases where the teacher was reprimanded because he or she "violated the students' privacy" after taking cell phones from students, while other teachers have been criticized for being too strict with students for not allowing them to do what they want during school hours.

We do not need more research!
The only thing needed is a competent staff . . .
who can work in peace without being
threatened, harassed or violated.

In Sweden – which has one of the most highly computerized educational systems in the world – results have plummeted regarding reading, writing and math skills. Today the system cannot afford to hire enough staff, no, and it has even been suggested that "tired of school" students will not be asked to finalize 2/3 of their secondary education. So the new tools do not impress – it just seems like we should be spending money on well-trained teachers with old teaching materials. Simultaneously there is a tendency for students in alternative schools such as Waldorf, Montessori and Reggio Emilia, to do slightly better and mature mentally faster; and it's very interesting because these schools do not use computers to the same degree as mainstream schools.

These new wireless devices are now flooding schools and homes. Examples of such sources of microwave radiation are wireless routers, computers with wireless network cards, wireless landline phones, tablets (like the iPad), mobile phones, etc. Several years ago evidence surfaced that exposure from electromagnetic fields can cause serious biological effects and health effects. Against this backdrop, many like myself protested, including parents, teachers and school staff in Köping as seen in Bärgslagsbladet (April 18) in 2012 under the headline "No to wireless at school."

Children are probably sensitive to pulsed microwave radiation from iPads and routers There are now numerous scientific studies that children are likely to be more vulnerable to pulsed microwave radiation than adults. New research shows, among other serious effects on behavior and learning ability, that there is general agreement among scientists that electromagnetic fields penetrate further into the brains of children than in adults because the skulls of children are thinner. There is also a broad consensus that children are more vulnerable to adverse effects from radiation because their bodies are developing, thus, by definition, more sensitive to environmental toxins. Children are not "little adults"!

The Council of Europe's Environment Committee has called for strong measures to protect the public against mobile phone radiation The World Health Organization in 2011 classified electromagnetic fields from wireless sources as possible carcinogens. In its Resolution No. 1815 from May 2011 the Council of Europe's Environment Committee recommended strong measures to protect the public against harmful effects of wireless radiation, including a ban on mobile phones and wireless internet in schools. It also wants to reduce the recommended maximal exposure level of mobile telephony sharply, all this completely in agreement with the Seletun declaration of 2010. In it, an international group of scientists urge on a stop to further expansion of wireless systems and require new guideline limits. In February 2010 The Seletun Scientific Panel published a resolution with a wide range of common positions and recommendations, based on a review of the then-available research on the health effects of electromagnetic fields. Since then there have been many more reports ...

The Swedish Radiation Safety Authority (SSM) misleads

Sometimes you see in the debate that someone – usually from a radiation safety organization – claims there is no danger and that "the radiation is so weak." Weak compared to what?, I wonder. Today there are children in radiation levels that could easily be 1,000,000,000,000,000,000 times higher than our natural background radiation. So how can the phrase "so weak" be justified? A child using a laptop to download from a wireless Internet connection is exposed to the same amount of radiation (about 1,000 µW/m2 and above) as if he/she were near a cellular base station (50-100 meters away). There are many parents who are not aware of this. The figures are not plucked from the air, but taken from readings in schools in Oslo by the Norwegian Post and Telecommunications Agency. Whether it's about base stations, wireless or cell phones, it is the same type of radiation we are talking about (in the range of 1-2.5 GHz).

Autism and ADHD-like behaviors

A group of researchers in California recently conducted a large study of mobile phone use in pregnant women. They looked at all the kids who were born in Denmark in a given year and interviewed the mothers about their mobile phone use during pregnancy. They also asked about the child's mobile usage and behavior. To the researchers' surprise it turned out that the mothers who had used mobile phones the most during pregnancy had the greatest risk of having children with behavioral difficulties.

It was about both autism and ADHD-like behaviors. The increase in risk was statistically significant. The risk also increased further if the child himself used a cell phone.

[Divan HA, Kheifets L, Obel C, Olsen J (2008) "Prenatal and postnatal exposure to cell phone use and behavioral problems in children", Epidemiology 2008; 19: 523-529.]

Symptoms: headache, abnormal fatigue and irritation Such a study might not be sufficient to conclude that electromagnetic fields are dangerous to children. German researchers wanted to measure the radiation dose that children and adolescents are exposed to in daily life. They asked about 3,000 children and young people in Bavaria to walk around carrying a dosimeter from morning to night. The dosimeters measured the radiation from cell phones, base stations and wireless networks. It turned out that the quarter of the children who were most exposed to radiation had more concentration problems at night than the rest of the kids. The same group also had more headaches and were more irritated than other young people. The results of the Bavarian study were again statistically significant. [Heinrich S, Thomas S, Heumann C, von Kries R, Radon K (2010) "Association between exposure to radiofrequency electromagnetic fields were assessed by dosimetry and acute symptoms in children and adolescents: a population-based cross-sectional study." [*Environmental Health* 2010, 9:75-83]

So the question is what mechanism can explain these symptoms in children and adolescents. Scientists Buchner & Eger in Germany measured levels of stress hormones in 60 residents in an area before a base station was erected. They were measured again after six months and again after one and a half years after the antenna became operational. It turned out that people had much higher levels of the stress hormones adrenaline and noradrenaline six months after the base station became operational, and after another year, the situation had not improved. Living with such constant stress to the body is obviously harmful to health. [Buchner K, Eger H, "Veränderung klinisch bedeutsamer Neurotransmitter unter dem Einfluss modulierter hochfrequenter Felder – Eine Langzeiterhebung unter lebensnahen Bedingungen", Umwelt – Medizin -Gesellschaft 2011: 24 : 44-57.]

Do not think this is just about the kids. Even fetuses are affected significantly and in a particularly scary way. Scientists

Jing, et al., of the Department of Public Health, Shandong University, China, have studied the impact of mobile phone radiation on pregnant rat fetuses. The researchers measured changes in both neuronal neurotransmitters and effects on antioxidant enzymes which protect our cells from oxidative stress. They conclude that mobile phone radiation during pregnancy resulted in damage to the fetal brains! They were born already brain-damaged. What mothers and fathers want that for their children?

[Jing J, Yuhua Z, Xiao- Qian Y, Rongping J, Dong- Mei G, Xi C, "The influence of microwave radiation from cellular phone on fetal rat brains," Electromag BiolMed 2012; 31:57-66.]

Students and teachers more and more frequently report abnormal fatigue in their working environment and you can not dismiss current suspicions that exposure from wireless networks can play a role in this. It is therefore important to ensure that wireless networks in kindergartens and schools are not causing significant and unnecessary risks for the health of our children and their teachers. Academically, the subject is not very complicated but for a layman can seem difficult to assess. The lack of knowledge today is due exclusively to the lack of research resources, not a lack of ideas, hypotheses, theories or interest.

The Precautionary Principle must be applied

Based on the above information the organization Citizens' Radiation Protection in Norway, http://www.folkets-stralevern.no/, has urged parents to sign a formal agreement where a parent does not consent to the exposure of their children to microwave radiation from wireless communication technology either in the classroom or indoors in general. As a parent, you are encouraged to require that the school/preschool exercises precautions to minimize radiation exposure and to demand wired solutions for data networking and telephony indoors. You are also encouraged to demand answers on who is responsible for the child if damaged by radiation exposure.

Time is not on our side. We must quickly decide how to proceed. In Sweden the choice seems to be having "artist types" running around in the community – wildly creative but totally impossible to put at the controls of an airplane or be responsible for the safety of a nuclear power plant. Alternatively should we have a population that is completely egalitarian, equipped with all the basics to work in our society? Will the next generation be capable at all of handling the different functions society requires? Do we want a society where we accept math, reading and writing difficulties that are solely due to the teaching handled by unauthorized personnel, through strange "apps" and in a computerized educational chaos?

But our Education Minister Jan Björklund has instead appointed an advisory committee of international experts called "the school commission". A new agency (an "educational research institute") is to be established to investigate these issues. In addition, Björklund intends to create a Swedish Education Council. He also talks about various new investigations and new reforms.

We do not need more research!

The only thing needed is a competent staff with good pay who can work in peace without being threatened, harassed or violated. Their work with students shall be in accordance with traditional effective educational models, with proven pedagogical aids, peace and quiet in class, concentration, joy, enthusiasm, teaching instead of gaming and mobile browsing, information tailored to each individual's ability, and demands on teachers and students in relation to future levels of responsibility. (However, during the public debate I have not heard or read anywhere that one should bet again on the school, the teachers, the educational content or the often poor school facilities and the salmonella-contaminated school lunches. But these are left unattended. Sounds like something out of a New Year's fun cabaret, right?)

Peter Kadhammar at the Swedish tabloid Aftonbladet notes in his excellent column from January 17, 2014, that" In the knowledge society literacy skills have been lost". As I have pointed out many times this has happened in spite of (!) the vast amounts of electronic gadgets introduced and now used in our Swedish schools. All iPads, WiFi, "surf the web pages", computer games, laptops, sending text messages during class, smart phones, etc., do not seem to have done their supposed job of teaching? Enough is enough. We need peace and quiet in the classroom. Put away the e-reader and mobile and kick out school politicians who want to spend money on unproven educational gadgets that are also probably merely health hazardous.

—Olle Johansson, Assoc. Professor and Asst. Professor in Neuroscience, Karolinska Institute, Stockholm.

Originally published by NewsVoice.se [Sweden], January 23, 2014: http://newsvoice.se/ 2014/01/23/ki-forskare-porta-skolpolitiker-som-vill-ge-formodat-halsofarliga-lasplattor-till-eleverna/.

Scientists Warn of Potential Serious Health Impacts of 5G

We the undersigned, more than 180 scientists and doctors from 36 countries, recommend a moratorium on the roll-out of the fifth generation, 5G, for telecommunication until potential hazards for human health and the environment have been fully investigated by scientists independent from industry. 5G will substantially increase exposure to radiofrequency electromagnetic fields (RF-EMF) on top of the 2G, 3G, 4G, WiFi, etc. for telecommunications already in place. RF-EMF has been proven to be harmful for humans and the environment.

5G leads to massive increase of mandatory exposure to wireless radiation

5G technology is effective only over short distance. It is poorly transmitted through solid material. Many new antennas will be required and full-scale implementation will result in antennas every 10 to 12 houses in urban areas, thus massively increasing mandatory exposure.

With "the ever more extensive use of wireless technologies," nobody can avoid to be exposed. Because on top of the increased number of 5G-transmitters (even within housing, shops and in hospitals) according to estimates, "10 to 20 billion connections" (to refrigerators, washing machines, surveillance cameras, self-driving cars and buses, etc.) will be parts of the Internet of Things. All these together can cause a substantial increase in the total, long term RF-EMF exposure to all EU citizens.

Harmful effects of RF-EMF exposure are already proven

Over 230 scientists from more than 40 countries have expressed their "serious concerns" regarding the ubiquitous and increasing exposure to EMF generated by electric and wireless devices already before the additional 5G roll-out. They refer to the fact that "numerous recent scientific publications have shown that EMF affects living organisms at levels well below most international and national guidelines." Effects include increased cancer risk, cellular stress, increase in harmful free radicals, genetic damages, structural and functional changes of the reproductive system, learning and memory deficits, neurological disorders, and negative impacts on general well-being in humans. Damage goes well beyond the human race, as there is growing evidence of harmful effects to both plants and animals.

After the scientists' appeal was written in 2015 additional research has convincingly confirmed serious health risks from RF-EMF fields from wireless technology. The world's largest study (25 million US dollar) National Toxicology Program (NTP), shows statistically significant increase in the incidence of brain and heart cancer in animals exposed to EMF below the ICNIRP (International Commission on Non-Ionizing Radiation Protection) guidelines followed by most countries. These results support results in human epidemiological studies on RF radiation and brain tumour risk. A large number of peer-reviewed scientific reports demonstrate harm to human health from EMFs.

The International Agency for Research on Cancer (IARC), the cancer agency of the World Health Organization (WHO), in 2011 concluded that EMFs of frequencies 30 KHz – 300 GHz are possibly carcinogenic to humans (Group 2B). However, new studies like the NTP study mentioned above and several epidemiological investigations including the latest studies on mobile phone use and brain cancer risks confirm that RF-EMF radiation is carcinogenic to humans.

The EUROPA EM-EMF Guideline 2016 states that "there is strong evidence that long-term exposure to certain EMFs is a risk factor for diseases such as certain cancers, Alzheimer's disease, and male infertility. ... Common EHS (electromagnetic hypersensitivity) symptoms include headaches, concentration difficulties, sleep problems, depression, lack of energy, fatigue, and flu-like symptoms."

An increasing part of the European population is affected by ill health symptoms that have for many years been linked to exposure to EMF and wireless radiation in the scientific literature. The International Scientific Declaration on EHS & multiple chemical sensitivity (MCS), Brussels 2015, declares that: "In view of our present scientific knowledge, we thereby stress all national and international bodies and institutions...to recognize EHS and MCS as true medical conditions which acting as sentinel diseases may create a major public health concern in years to come worldwide i.e. in all the countries implementing unrestricted use of electromagnetic field-based wireless technologies and marketed chemical substances ... Inaction is a cost to society and is not an option anymore ... we unanimously acknowledge this serious hazard to public health ... that major primary prevention measures are adopted and prioritized, to face this worldwide pan-epidemic in perspective."

Precautions

The Precautionary Principle (UNESCO) was adopted by EU 2005: "When human activities may lead to morally unacceptable harm that is scientifically plausible but uncertain, actions shall be taken to avoid or diminish that harm."

Resolution 1815 (Council of Europe, 2011): "Take all reasonable measures to reduce exposure to electromagnetic fields, especially to radio frequencies from mobile phones, and particularly the exposure to children and young people who seem to be most at risk from head tumours...Assembly strongly recommends that the ALARA (as low as reasonably achievable) principle is applied, covering both the so-called thermal effects and the athermic [non-thermal] or biological effects of electromagnetic emissions or radiation" and to "improve risk-assessment standards and quality."

The Nuremberg code (1949) applies to all experiments on humans, thus including the roll-out of 5G with new, higher RF-EMF exposure. All such experiments: "should be based on previous knowledge (e.g., an expectation derived from animal experiments) that justifies the experiment. No experiment should be conducted, where there is an a priori reason to believe that death or disabling injury will occur; except, perhaps, in those experiments where the experimental physicians also serve as subjects." (Nuremberg code pts 3-5). Already published scientific studies show that there is "a priori reason to believe" in real health hazards.

The European Environment Agency (EEA) is warning for "Radiation risk from everyday devices" in spite of the radiation being below the WHO/ICNIRP standards. EEA also concludes: "There are many examples of the failure to use the precautionary principle in the past, which have resulted in serious and often irreversible damage to health and environments...harmful exposures can be widespread before there is both 'convincing' evidence of harm from long-term exposures, and biological understanding [mechanism] of how that harm is caused."

"Safety guidelines" protect industry—not health

The current ICNIRP "safety guidelines" are obsolete. All proofs of harm mentioned above arise although the radiation is below the ICNIRP "safety guidelines." Therefore new safety standards are necessary. The reason for the misleading guidelines is that "conflict of interest of ICNIRP members due to their relationships with telecommunications or electric companies undermine the impartiality that should govern the regulation of Public Exposure Standards for non-ionizing radiation ... To evaluate cancer risks it is necessary to include scientists with competence in medicine, especially oncology."

The current ICNIRP/WHO guidelines for EMF are based on the obsolete hypothesis that "The critical effect of RF-EMF exposure relevant to human health and safety is heating of exposed tissue." However, scientists have proven that many different kinds of illnesses and harms are caused without heating ("nonthermal effect") at radiation levels well below ICNIRP guidelines.

We urge EU:

1) To take all reasonable measures to halt the 5G RF-EMF expansion until independent scientists can assure that 5G and the total radiation levels caused by RF-EMF (5G together with 2G, 3G, 4G, and WiFi) will not be harmful for EU-citizens, especially infants, children and pregnant women, as well as the environment
2) To recommend that all EU countries, especially their radiation safety agencies, follow Resolution 1815 and inform citizens, including, teachers and physicians, about health risks from RF-EMF radiation, how and why to avoid wireless communication, particularly in/near e.g., daycare centers, schools, homes, workplaces, hospitals and elderly care.
3) To appoint immediately, without industry influence, an EU task force of independent, truly impartial EMF-and-health scientists with no conflicts of interest1 to re-evaluate the health risks and:
    a) To decide about new, safe "maximum total exposure standards" for all wireless communication within EU.
    b) To study the total and cumulative exposure affecting EU-citizens.
    c) To create rules that will be prescribed/enforced within the EU about how to avoid exposure exceeding new EU "maximum total exposure standards" concerning all kinds of EMFs in order to protect citizens, especially infants, children and pregnant women.

4) To prevent the wireless/telecom industry through its lobbying organizations from persuading EU officials to make decisions about further propagation of RF radiation including 5G in Europe.
5) To favor and implement wired digital telecommunication instead of wireless.

We expect an answer from you no later than October 31, 2017 to the two first mentioned signatories about what measures you will take to protect the EU-inhabitants against RF-EMF and especially 5G radiation. This appeal and your response will be publicly available.

Respectfully submitted,

Rainer Nyberg, EdD, Professor Emeritus (Åbo Akademi), Vasa, Finland

Lennart Hardell, MD, PhD, Professor (assoc) Department of Oncology, Faculty of Medicine and Health, University Hospital, Örebro, Sweden

Signatories to Scientists' 5G Appeal

The full list of signatories to the 5G Appeal would go on for pages. Those that follow are from the United States.

Note: The endorsements are personal and not necessarily supported by the affiliated universities or organizations. Updated with new Signatories: September 15, 2017.

David O. Carpenter, MD, Director, Institute for Health and the Environment, A Collaborating Centre of the World Health Organization, University at Albany, Rensselaer, NY

Barry Castleman, ScD, Environmental Consultant, Garrett Park, MD.

Devra Davis, PhD, MPH, Visiting Prof. Medicine, Hebrew

University, Hadassah Medical Center & Ondokuz Mayis University, Medical School (Turkey); Pres., Environmental Health Trust, Teton Village, WY

Paul Doyon, MA, MAT, EMRS, Independent Researcher, Doyon Independent Research, CA

Arthur Firstenberg, BA, EMF researcher and author, president Cellular Phone Task Force, New York

Beatrice A. Golomb, MD, PhD, Professor of Medicine, University of California, San Diego, CA

Peter F. Infante, PhD, Managing Member, Peter F. Infante Consulting, LLC, VA

Toril H. Jelter, MD, MDI Wellness Center, CA

Elizabeth Kelley, MA, Electromagnetic Safety Alliance, Tucson, AZ

Henry Lai, PhD, Professor Emeritus, University of Washington, Seattle, WA

B. Blake Levitt, medical/science journalist, former New York Times contributor, EMF researcher and author

Trevor G Marshall, ME, PhD, Director, Autoimmunity Research Foundation, CA

Ronald Melnick, PhD, Senior Toxicologist, (Retired RF-section leader) US National Toxicology Program, National Institute of Environmental Health Sciences

L. Lloyd Morgan, Senior Research Fellow, Environmental Health Trust, Board Member, International EMF Alliance (IEMFA), CA

S. M. J. Mortazavi, PhD, Professor of Medical Physics, Visiting Scientist, Fox Chase Cancer Center, Philadelphia, PA

Joel M. Moskowitz, PhD, Director, Center for Family and Community Health, School of Public Health, University of California, Berkeley, CA

Martin Pall, BA, PhD, Professor Emeritus (Biochemistry and basic medicine), Pullman, WA

Jerry L. Phillips, PhD, Exec. Director, Excel Centers, Professor Attendant, Department of Chemistry & Biochemistry,

University of Colorado, Colorado Springs, CO
Camilla R. G. Rees, MBA, Health Researcher, Author, "The Wireless Elephant in the Room," CEO, Wide Angle Health, Sr. Policy Advisor, National Institute for Science, Law & Public Policy, NY
Cindy Sage, MA, Sage Associates, Co-editor, *BioInitiative 2007* and *BioInitiative 2012*, Santa Barbara, CA
Eugene Sobel, PhD, Professor (Retired), University of Southern California School of Medicine, CA
John G. West, MD, Director of Surgery, Breastlink, CA
Cindy Russell, MD, Founding Member, Physicians for Safe Technology, CA

Source: EMF Alliance. For a complete list of the signatories, go to iemfa.org/news/ and click on the link to the Appeal for 5G Moratorium.

Addendum: On May 14, 2018, signator Arthur Firstenberg, representing the Global Union Against Radiation Deployment from Space (GUARDS), had an article, "Planetary Emergency," published by the Cellular Phone Task Force regarding the further intrusion of 5G technology. He wrote, in part:

"On March 29, 2018, the Federal Communications Commission gave its approval to SpaceX's plan to launch an unprecedented 4,425 satellites into low orbit around the earth. And that's only the beginning. SpaceX has applied to the FCC to increase the number of satellites to 12,000 in order to provide "ultrafast, lag-free Internet" to every square inch of the earth. 5G from space."

To read the entire piece online, go to: cellphonetaskforce.org/planetary-emergency.

Appendix V

Exposing the Industry's Lies About Cell Phone Radiation

The World Health Organization declared in May 2011 that cell phone use may cause brain cancer after 10 years for an average use of only 30 minutes per day.

EVERY cell phone sold in the U.S. comes with a government-required safety warning (hidden in the legal fine print that no one reads) that using or carrying a phone directly against the body may expose the user to more microwave radiation than allowed by federal safety limits.

The cell phone industry exerts powerful influence with their wide spread and intense lobbying of our state and federal elected representatives and regulatory agency officials. They intimidate scientists to manipulate their cell phone exposure research findings to ensure they show no negative health risks. Their well-paid PR firms "spin" the science and provide "whitewashed" press releases to media assuring us that cell phones are safe and those who say otherwise are fear mongers and conspiracy theorists.

Their deception of the American people in the name of corporate profit-making must stop!

Here are just a few of their lies and the facts they are trying to hide:

Reprinted with permission of Consumers for Safe Phones. consumers4safephones.com.

LIE: The majority of studies that have been published in scientific journals around the world show that wireless phones do not pose a health risk.

LIE: If cell phones were causing brain tumors, with so many people using them, we should be seeing an increase in brain tumor incidence, and we are not.

LIE: The Federal Communications Commission (FCC) requires testing of all cell phones to ensure they do not exceed the federal exposure standard; the FCC declares that phones complying with this standard are safe.

LIE: The FCC's exposure standard protects even children from the emissions from cell phones.

LIE: The World Health Organization, National Cancer Institute, and American Cancer Society all declare that cell phones are safe.

TRUTH: *When one removes the industry-funded studies, the overwhelming weight of the evidence shows there IS a significant health risk from the exposure to microwave radiation emitted by cell phones and other wireless devices.*

TRUTH: *There is a longer latency period for brain tumors. Cell phones have only been widely used in the U.S. for two decades. Despite this, a recently released study shows an increase in brain tumors in 3 major cancer registries in the United States. The increase seen is in the frontal and temporal lobes, the two regions closest to where a cell phone is typically held.*

TRUTH: *FCC requires testing to ensure cell phones meet the federal exposure standard, but the exposure standard used is set so high that it only takes into account the tissue burning effect of the microwave radiation. Hundreds of published studies show health effects that cause reduced fertility, cardiac incidents, anxiety, insomnia, reduced concentration, exhaustion, DNA damage and increased risk of ADHD in children AT LEVELS THOUSANDS OF TIMES BELOW THE FCC STANDARD.*

TRUTH: *Children's brains absorb up to 2 times as much microwave radiation from cell phones as adult brains; the FCC standard does NOT protect children and most teens as their exposure standard is based upon an enormous 220-pound, 6'2" man.*

TRUTH: *These agencies do NOT declare that cell phones are safe. In 2011, the World Health Organization (WHO) classified cell phone radiation exposure as a 2B carcinogen placing it in the same health risk category as lead and DDT. NCI's website states, "More research is needed because cell phone technology and how people use cell phones have been changing rapidly." And, from the ACS website, "It is important that the possible risk of cell phone exposure continue to be researched using strong study methods, especially with regard to use by children and longer term use."*

OTHER FACTS THE CELL PHONE INDUSTRY DOES NOT WANT YOU TO KNOW:

- According to a 2011 Pew Research report, 66% of all U.S. children acquire a cell phone before the age of 7 and 87% of teens sleep with them under their pillows while connected to the network emitting microwave radiation into their heads throughout the night.
- *2012 Government Accountability Office (GAO) study concluded,* ***"Some consumers may use mobile phones against the body, which FCC does not currently test, and could result in RF energy exposure higher than the FCC limit."***

References

Adey, W.R. "Biological Effects of Electromagnetic Fields," *Journal of Cellular Biochemistry*, 51, No. 4 (April 1993).

Albarazi, Hannah. "Cellphone Radiation Exposure Fact Sheet Draft Released By California Health Officials," CBS SFBayArea, March 2, 2017. Retrieved 2018 from http://sanf7rancisco.cbslocal.com/2017/03/02/cellphone-radiation-exposure-fact-sheet-draft-released-by-california-health-officials/.

Alleyne, Richard. "Mobile phones can cause brain tumours, [Italian] court rules," *The Telegraph*, October 19, 2012. Retrieved 2018 from https://www.telegraph.co.uk/news/9619514/Mobile-phones-can-cause-brain-tumours-court-rules.html.

Associated Press. "Hang up on cancer-cell phone link," *Las Vegas Review Journal*, February 3-4, 2018.

Associated Press. "Wisconsin Farmer Wins Stray Voltage Case Against Xcel Energy," *US News*, August 7, 2017. Retrieved 2017 from https://www.usnews.com/news/best-states/wisconsin/articles/2017-08-07/wisconsin-farmer-wins-stray-voltage-case-against-xcel-energy.

Austrian Medical Association. "Guideline of the Austrian Medical Association for the diagnosis and treatment of EMF-related health problems and illnesses (EMF syndrome)," Austrian Medical Association's EMF Working Group, March, 2012.

Retrieved 2018 from www.vagbrytaren.org/Guideline%20%20AG-EMF.pdf.

Autism Speaks; https://www.autismspeaks.org.

BabyTechSummit.com. "ThermoSafer," 2017. Retrieved 2018 from awards.babytechsummit.com/bestof2017/ thermosafer/.

Banaszkiewicz, Tadeusz. "Evolution of Pesticide Use," *Influence of the Pesticide Dump on the Environment: Contemporary Problems of Management and Environmental Protection*, Poland: Uniwersytet Warmińsko-Mazurski w Olsztynie, Volume 5, 2010; (Chapter 1) 7-18. Retrieved 2018 from www.uwm.edu.pl/environ/vol05/vol_05_chapter01.pdf.

Barbalace, Roberta C. "A Brief History of Asbestos Use and Associated Health Risks," EnvironmentalChemistry.com. October, 2004. Retrieved February 24, 2018, from https://EnvironmentalChemistry.com/yogi/environmental/asbestoshistory2004.html.

Barrett, Julia R., MS, ELS. "An Uneven Path Forward: The History of Methylmercury Toxicity Research," *Environmental Health Perspectives*, August, 2010; 118(8): A352.

Barsam, Tayebeh, Mohammad Reza Monazzam, Ali Akbar Haghdoost, Mohammad Reza Ghotbi, and Somayeh Farhang Dehghan. "Effect of extremely low frequency electromagnetic field exposure on sleep quality in high voltage substations," *Iranian Journal of Environmental Health, Science & Engineering*, published online November 30, 2012; 9(1): 15. doi: 10.1186/1735-2746-9-15.

Bates, Clive, and Andy Rowell. "The truth about the tobacco industry . . . in its own words," Action on Smoking and Health, June 25, 1998. Retrieved 2018 from http://www.who.int/tobacco/media/en/TobaccoExplained.pdf.

Bauer, Brent A., MD. "What is BPA, and what are the concerns about BPA?" Mayo Clinic, [Undated]. Retrieved 2018 from https://www.mayoclinic.org/healthy-lifestyle/nutrition-and-healthy-eating/expert-answers/bpa/faq-20058331.

BBC News. "Child warning over mobile phones," January 11, 2005. Retrieved 2017 from http://news.bbc.co.uk/2/hi/health/4163003.stm.

BBC News. "Wisconsin company Three Square Market to microchip employees," July 24, 2017. Retrieved 2018 from http://www.bbc.com/news/world-us-canada-40710051.

Becker, Rachel. "Driving and texting is much more likely to kill you than cell phone radiation. So why are we still talking about the radiation?" The Verge, April 5, 2018. Retrieved 2018 from theverge.com/2018/4/5/17202600/cell-phone-radiation-cancer-national-toxicology-program-wireless-health-effect-fears.

Bell, G.B., A.A. Marino and A.L. Chesson. "Frequency-specific responses in the human brain caused by electromagnetic fields," *Journal of Neurological Sciences*,1994; 123:26–32.

Belluz, Julia. "A concerning new study links miscarriages to cell phone radiation. How worried should we be? Non-ionizing radiation may have more of a biological effect than we thought," Vox Media, February 15, 2018. Retrieved 2018 from https://www.vox.com/science-and-health/2018/2/15/17008482/cellphones-cancer-miscarriage-health.

Belyaev, I. "Evidence for Disruption by Modulation: Role of Physical and Biological Variables in Bioeffects of Non-Thermal Microwaves for Reproducibility, Cancer Risk and Safety Standards," *BioInitiative 2012: A Rationale for a Biologically-based Public Exposure Standard for Electromagnetic Fields (ELF and RF),* C. Sage and D. O. Carpenter (editors). Retrieved 2017 from http://www.bioinitiative.org/.

Blackman, C. "Evidence for Disruption by the Modulating Signal," *BioInitiative 2007: A Rationale for a Biologically-based Public Exposure Standard for Electromagnetic Fields (ELF and RF),* C. Sage and D. O. Carpenter (editors). Retrieved 2017 from http://www.bioinitiative.org/.

Blank, Martin, PhD, and Reba M. Goodman, PhD. "Electromagnetic fields and health: DNA-based dosimetry," *Electromagnetic Biology and Medicine*, June 7, 2012.

Blum, Deborah. "The Formaldehyde Conspiracy," *Wired*, October 10, 2012. Retrieved 2018 from https://www.wired.com/2012/10/the-formaldehyde-conspiracy/.

Borentstein, Seth, and Lauran Neergaard. "Cancer from Cellphones? New Studies Say No Need to Hang Up," *Wireless Week*, February 5, 2018. Retrieved 2018 from https://www.wirelessweek.com/news/2018/02/cancer-cellphones-new-studies-say-no-need-hang.

Borio, Gene. "Tobacco history—headlines," Notobacco Center, Tripod.com, 2001. Retrieved 2018 from http://notabaco.tripod.com/notabacocenter/id4.html.

Borio, Gene. "Tobacco Timeline," Tobacco News and Information, 2001. Retrieved 2018 from http://archive.tobacco.org/History/Tobacco_History.html.

Borio, Gene. "Tobacco Timeline: The Twentieth Century 1900-1949—The Rise of the Cigarette," SCRIBD.com, 2003. Retrieved 2018 from https://www.scribd.com/document/328812194/Tobacco-Timeline.

Bradford, Alina. "How Blue LEDs Affect Sleep," Live Science, February 26, 2016. Retrieved 2018 from https://www.livescience.com/53874-blue-light-sleep.html.

Brunner, Jordan, and Emma Kohse. "Supreme Court Grants Cert in Carpenter v. United States: An Overview," Lawfare, June 6, 2017. Retrieved 2018 from https://www.lawfareblog.com/supreme-court-grants-cert-carpenter-v-united-states-overview.

Burrell, Lloyd. *EMF Practical Guide: The Simple Science of Protecting Yourself, Healing Chronic Inflammation, and Living a Naturally Healthy Life in Our Toxic Electromagnetic World*. Royan, France: ElectricSense, 2019.

Caliendo, Heather. "Food Safety: History of BPA," *Packaging Digest*, June 28, 2012. Retrieved 2018 from http://www.packagingdigest.com/food-safety/history-bpa.

California Department of Public Health, Division of Environmental and Occupational Disease Control. "How to Reduce Exposure to Radiofrequency Energy from Cell Phones," December 22, 2017. Retrieved 2018 from https://www.cdph.ca.gov/Programs/CCDPHP/DEODC/.

Calvente, I., M.F. Fernandez, J. Villalba, N. Olea, M.I. Nunez MI. "Exposure to electromagnetic fields (non-ionizing radiation) and its relationship with childhood leukemia: a systematic review," *Science of the Total Environment*, July 15, 2010, 408(16):3062-9. doi: 10.1016/j.scitotenv.2010.03.039. Epub May 7, 2010.

Campbell, Charlie. "How China Is Using 'Social Credit Scores' to Reward and Punish Its Citizens," *Time*, Jan. 17, 2019. Retrieved January 2020 from https://time.com/collection/davos-2019/5502592/china-social-credit-score/.

Carlo, George, and Martin Schram. *Cell Phones: Invisible Hazards in the Wireless Age*. New York, NY: Avalon, 2001.

Carlo, George. "Invisible Hazards in the Wireless Age: The Research & The Recommendations" [Biographical Statement], International Electromagnetic Fields Alliance, [Undated]. Retrieved 2018 from http://www.iemfa.org/wp-content/pdf/George%20Carlo2.pdf.

Carlo, George. "The Wireless Industry Is Committing Scientific Fraud" [Video], Electromagnetic Radiation Health Effects, March 23, 2014. Retrieved 2018 from https://www.youtube.com/watch?v=vsv0k5zvRXA.

Carney, Matthew. "South Korean Children Seek Help at Digital Detox Boot Camp," ABC News Australia, September 15, 2015. Retrieved 2018 from http://www.abc.net.au/news/2015-09-13/south-korean-children-seek-help-at-digital-detox-boot-camp/6769766.

Carpenter, D.O., and C. Sage (editors). *BioInitiative 2012—A Rationale for a Biologically-based Public Exposure Standard for Electromagnetic Fields (ELF and RF),* BioInitiative Report, Rensselaer, NY: University at Albany, 2012. Retrieved 2017 from http://www.bioinitiative.org/.

Carson, Rachel. *Silent Spring*, Boston, MA: Houghton Mifflin Co., 1962.

Center for Responsive Politics. "Electric Utilities," OpenSecrets.org, [Undated]. Retrieved 2018 from https://www.opensecrets.org/industries/indus.php?Ind=E08.

Center for Responsive Politics. "Lobbying Data Summary, 2019," OpenSecrets.org, [Undated]. Retrieved February 19, 2020, from https://www.opensecrets.org/federal-lobbying/summary.

Center for Responsive Politics. "Revolving Door," OpenSecrets.org, [Undated]. https://www.opensecrets.org/revolving/.

Center for Responsive Politics. "Top Contributors to political campaigns from the oil and gas industry, 2017-2018" [Summary], OpenSecrets.org, [Undated]. Retrieved 2018 from https://www.opensecrets.org/industries/indus.php?ind=E01.

Central Brain Tumor Registry of the United States; cbtrus.org.

Chamberlin, Jamie. "Smart glasses: Driver distraction or safety tool?" *American Psychological Association*, March 2014, Vol. 45, No. 3. Retrieved 2018 from http://www.apa.org/monitor/2014/03/smart-glasses.aspx.

Chen, Brian X. "In an Era of 'Smart' Things, Sometimes Dumb Stuff Is Better," *The New York Times*, February 21, 2018. Retrieved 2018 from https://www.nytimes.com/2018/02/21/technology/personaltech/smart-things-dumb-stuff.html.

Chen, Heather. "Asia's smartphone addiction," BBC News, Singapore, September 7, 2015. Retrieved 2018 from http://www.bbc.com/news/world-asia-33130567.

Cherry, Neil. Re: "Cancer incidence near radio and television transmitters in Great Britain. II: All high power transmitters, Dolk et al., 1997 a,b in *American Journal of Epidemiology*, 145(1):1-9 and 10-17. Comment in *American Journal of Epidemiology*, 153(2) (January 15, 2001): 204-205.

Cherry, Neil. "Probable health effects associated with mobile base stations in communities: the need for health studies." Canterbury, NZ: Lincoln University, Human Sciences Department, June 8, 2000.

Coldewey, Devin. "NIH study links cell phone radiation to cancer in male rats," TechCrunch, February 2, 2018. Retrieved 2018 from https://techcrunch.com/2018/02/02/ nih-study-links-cell-phone-radiation-to-cancer-in-male-rats/.

Collins, Tim. "Google and Amazon really DO want to spy on you: Patent reveals future versions of their voice assistants will record your conversations to sell you products," Consumer Watchdog, Dec. 15, 2017. Retrieved January 2020 from https://www.consumerwatchdog.org/privacy-technology/google-and-amazon-really-do-want-spy-you-patent-reveals-future-versions-their.

Concept Films. *Smoking and Health: The Need to Know* [Corporate Communication, 1972], UCSF Library: Truth Initiative—Inspiring Tobacco-Free Lives, June 16, 2006. Retrieved 2018 from industrydocumentslibrary.ucsf.edu/tobacco/ docs/#id=lkjy0104.

Consumers for Safe Phones. "Exposing the Industry's Lies About Cell Phone Radiation," [Undated]. Retrieved 2017 from http://consumers4safephones.com.

Consumers for Safe Phones. "FCC's Cell Phone Testing Dummy Is Larger Than 97% of All Cell Phone Users," November 27, 2011. Retrieved 2017 from http://consumers4safephones.com/fccs-cell-phone-testing-dummy-is-larger-than-97-of-all-cell-phone-users/.

Cooper, Anderson (host). "Is Your Cell Phone Safe? Cooper and Gupta Discuss Cell Phone Safety" [Television Newscast], CNN Press Room, May 31, 2011. Retrieved 2017 from http://cnnpressroom.blogs.cnn.com/2011/05/31/anderson-cooper-and-dr-sanjay-gupta-discuss-cell-phone-safety/.

Cooper, Carleigh. *Cell Phones and The Dark Deception: Find Out What You're Not Being Told . . . And Why*, Grandville, MI: Premier Advantage Publishing, 2009.

Crichton, Danny. "Ultra-fast 5G wireless service declared national security priority by White House," TechCrunch.com, December 19, 2017. Retrieved 2018 from https://techcrunch.com/2017/

12/19/ultra-fast-5g-wireless-service-declared-national-security-priority-by-white-house/.

Cummings, K.M., C.P. Morley, and A. Hyland. "Failed promises of the cigarette industry and its effect on consumer misperceptions about the health risks of smoking," *Tobacco Control* 2002;11(Suppl I):i110–i117.

Cummings, K. Michael, and Robert N. Proctor. "The Changing Public Image of Smoking in the United States: 1964–2014," *Cancer Epidemiology, Biomarkers & Prevention*, January, 2014; 23(1): 32–36. doi: 10.1158/1055-9965.EPI-13-0798.

Cuthbertson, Anthony. "Amazon Admits Employees Listen to Alexa Conversations," *Independent*, April 11, 2019. Retrieved January 2020 from https://www.independent.co.uk/life-style/gadgets-and-tech/news/amazon-alexa-echo-listening-spy-security-a8865056.html.

Davis, Devra, PhD, MPH. *Disconnect: The Truth About Cell Phone Radiation*, New York, NY: Environmental Health Trust, 2013.

DeBaun, Daniel T., and Ryan DeBaun. *Radiation Nation: Fallout of Modern Technology—Your Complete Guide to EMF Protection & Safety: The Proven Health Risks of Electromagnetic Radiation (EMF) & What to Do Protect Yourself & Family*, Icaro Publishing, March 20, 2017.

Deen, Thalif. "U.S. Lags Far Behind in Banning Dental Health Hazard," Inter Press Service, July 31, 2017. Retrieved 2018 from http://www.ipsnews.net/2017/07/us-lags-far-behind-banning-dental-health-hazard/.

Divan, H.A., L. Kheifets, C. Obel, J. Olsen. "Prenatal and postnatal exposure to cell phone use and behavioral problems in children," *Epidemiology*, 2008; 19: 523-529.

Doheny, Kathleen. "Autism Cases on the Rise; Reason for Increase a Mystery," WebMD, [Undated]. Retrieved 2017 from https://www.webmd.com/brain/autism/searching-for-answers/autism-rise.

Dokoupil, Tony. "Is the Internet Making Us Crazy? What the New Research Says," *Newsweek*, July 9, 2012. Retrieved 2018 from http://www.newsweek.com/internet-making-us-crazy-what-new-research-says-65593.

Dunckley, Victoria L., MD. "Electronic Screen Syndrome: An Unrecognized Disorder?" *Psychology Today*, July 23, 2012. Retrieved 2017 from https://www.psychologytoday.com/blog/mental-wealth/201207/electronic-screen-syndrome-unrecognized-disorder.

Eberhardt, J.L., B.R. Persson, A.E. Brun, L.G. Salford, and L.O. Malmgren. "Blood-brain barrier permeability and nerve cell damage in rat brain 14 and 28 days after exposure to microwaves from GSM mobile phones," *Electromagnetic Biology and Medicine*, 27 (3) (2008): 215-229; DOI:10.1080153637080234403 7.

Eby, Michael. "EMF and Public Health," EC&M, September 1, 2006. Retrieved 2018 from http://www.ecmweb.com/content/emf-and-public-health.

Eggleston, D.W. "Effect of Dental Amalgam and Nickel Alloys on T-lymphocytes: Preliminary Report," May 5, 1984; 51(5): 617, 619.

Eggleston, D.W., and M. Nylander. "The Correlation of Dental Amalgam with Mercury in Brain Tissue." *Journal of Prosthetic Dentistry*, December, 1987; 58: 704-707.

Elgan, Mike. "Uh-oh: Silicon Valley is building a Chinese-style social credit system," Fast Company, August 2019. Retrieved January 2020 from https://www.fastcompany.com/90394048/uh-oh-silicon-valley-is-building-a-chinese-style-social-credit-system.

Eliopoulos C., J. Klein, M.K. Phan et al. "Hair concentrations of nicotine and cotinine in women and their newborn infants." *JAMA*, 1994; 271: 621–3.

EM Radiation Research Trust. "News Media Nix NTP Cancer Study; 'Don't Believe the Hype': Are More People Getting Brain Tumors? GBMs, the Most Virulent Type, Are Rising," May 31, 2016; updated June 2, 2016. Retrieved 2018 from http://www.radiationresearch.org/news/news-media-nix-ntp-

phone-cancer-study-dont-believe-the-hype/.
Environmental Health Trust. "Advice of Cyprus National Committee on Environment and Children's Health" [Video], posted to YouTube by EHT, January 3, 2016. Retrieved 2018 from https://www.youtube.com/watch?v=H43IKNjTvRM.
Environmental Health Trust. "Database of Worldwide Policies on Cell Phones, Wireless and Health," [Undated]. Retrieved 2018 from https://ehtrust.org/policy/international-policy-actions-on-wireless/.
Environmental Working Group. "Dioxin Timeline—EPA'S Dioxin Assessment: No Safety Standard After Nearly Three Decades of Work," July 13, 2010. Retrieved 2018 from https://www.ewg.org/about-us#.WpYDxHxG1lc.
European Environment Agency. "Health risks from mobile phone radiation—why the experts disagree, October 12, 2011. Retrieved 2018 from https://www.eea.europa.eu/highlights/health-risks-from-mobile-phone.
Fairfield, Joshua A. T. *Owned: Property, Privacy and the New Digital Serfdom*, New York, NY: Cambridge University Press, 2017.
Federal Communications Commission, United States of America; https://www.fcc.gov/.
Federal Communications Commission. "New National Wireless Tower Siting Policies," FCC Fact Sheet, April 23, 1996. Retrieved 2018 from wireless.fcc.gov/fact1.pdf.
Feltman, Rachel. "Do Cell Phones Cause Cancer? Don't Believe the Hype." *Washington Post*, May 27, 2016. Retrieved 2018 from washingtonpost.com/news/speaking-of-science/wp/ 2016/05/27/do-cellphones-cause-cancer-dont-believe-the-hype/.
Firstenberg, Arthur. *The Invisible Rainbow, A History of Electricity and Life*. Santa Fe, NM: AGB Press, 2017.
Firstenberg, Arthur. "Planetary Emergency," Cellular Phone Task Force, May 14, 2018. Retrieved 2018 from http://www.cellphonetaskforce.org/planetary-emergency/.

Firstenberg, Arthur. "Report on National Toxicology Program's Cell Phone Study," April 12, 2018. Retrieved 2018 from http://www.cellphonetaskforce.org/wp-content/uploads/2018/04/NTP-analysis.pdf.

Foresman, Chris. "Wireless survey: 91% of Americans use cell phones," Ars Technica, March 24, 2010. Retrieved 2018 from https://arstechnica.com/tech-policy/2010/03/ wireless-survey-91-of-americans-have-cell-phones/.

Forum News Service. "$6.3M judgment in Minnesota dairy farm's stray voltage suit upheld," *Twin Cities Pioneer Press*, February 22, 2016. Retrieved 2017 from https://www.twincities.com/2016/02/22/6-3m-judgment-in-minnesota-dairy-farms-stray-voltage-suit-upheld/.

Fowler, Geoffrey A. "It's the middle of the night. Do you know who your iPhone is talking to?," *Washington Post*, May 28, 2019. Retrieved January 2020 from https://www.washingtonpost.com/technology/2019/05/28/its-middle-night-do-you-know-who-your-iphone-is-talking/.

Fowler, Geoffrey A. "No secrets at home anymore. Now Amazon's Alexa is spying on us," Stuff.co.nz, May 7, 2019. Retrieved January 2020 from https://www.stuff.co.nz/business/world/112528222/no-secrets-at-home-anymore-now-amazons-alexa-is-spying-on-us.

Fowler, Tristan. "A Brief History of Lead Regulation," *Science Progress*, October 21, 2008. Retrieved 2018 from https://scienceprogress.org/2008/10/a-brief-history-of-lead-regulation/.

Freeman, David. "New Smart Diaper Uses Wireless Sensor To Alert Parents When Baby Needs Changing," *Huffington Post*, February 12, 2014. Retrieved 2018 from https://www.huffingtonpost.com/2014/02/12/smart-diaper-wireless-sensor-alert-baby_n_4768837.html.

Frey, A., et al. "Neural Function and Behavior: Defining the Relationship," The New York Academy of Sciences [Online], February 1975. Retrieved June 9, 2017, from http://onlinelibrary.wiley.com/doi/10.1111/j.1749-6632.1975.tb36019.x/abstract.

Frey, A. "Studies of the blood-brain barrier: Preliminary findings and discussion," *Radio Science*, November 1979; DOI: 10.1029/RS014i06Sp00349. Retrieved 2018 from http://onlinelibrary.wiley.com/doi/10.1029/RS014i06Sp00349/abstract.

Fruhlinger, Josh. "The Mirai botnet explained: How teen scammers and CCTV cameras almost brought down the internet," CSO Online, March 9, 2018. Retrieved January 2020 from https://www.csoonline.com/article/3258748/the-mirai-botnet-explained-how-teen-scammers-and-cctv-cameras-almost-brought-down-the-internet.html.

Furniere, Andy. "Belgium bans sale of mobile phones designed for children," *Flanders Today* [Belgium], March 21, 2018. Retrieved 2018 from http://www.flanderstoday.eu/innovation/belgium-bans-sale-mobile-phones-designed-children.

Gandhi, Om P., L. Lloyd Morgan, Alvaro Augusto de Salles, Yueh-Ying Han, Ronald B. Herberman, and Devra Lee Davis. "Exposure Limits: The Underestimation of Absorbed Cell Phone Radiation, Especially in Children," *Electromagnetic Biology and Medicine*, March 31, 2012; 31(1):34-51. doi: 10.3109/15368378.2011.622827. Epub October 14, 2011.

Gazdecki, Andrew. "Smart Technology and the Internet of Things," BiznessAPPS.com, [Undated]. Retrieved 2018 from https://www.biznessapps.com/blog/smart-technology-and-the-internet-of-things/.

Gemayel, Sabine El (director). *Generation Zapped* [Documentary Film]. United States, 2017.

Gertz, Bill. "'Social credit score': China set to roll out 'Orwellian' mass surveillance tool," *The Washington Times*, Dec. 9, 2019. Retrieved January 2020 from https://www.washingtontimes.com/ news/ 2019/dec/9/social-credit-system-china-mass-surveillance-tool-/.

Gibson, Pamela R. "The Hidden Marginalization of Persons with Environmental Sensitivities," *Ecopsychology*, Vol. 8, No. 2, published online June 27, 2016. Retrieved 2018 from https://www.liebertpub.com/doi/full/10.1089/eco.2016.0003.

Gillette, Britt. "Will Artificial Intelligence Create Pathway To The Antichrist?," Prophecy News Watch, Nov. 19, 2019. Retrieved January 2020 from https://www.prophecynewswatch.com/article.cfm?recent_news_id=3610#QUFHUABSoVj1W5pv.99.

Gilson, Dave. "Who Owns Congress? A Campaign Cash Seating Chart," *Mother Jones*, September/October 2010. Retrieved 2018 from https://www.motherjones.com/politics/2010/10/congress-corporate-sponsors/.

Gittleman, Ann Louise. *Zapped: Why Your Cell Phone Shouldn't be Your Alarm Clock and 1,268 Ways to Outsmart the Hazards of Electronic Pollution*, New York, NY: McGraw-Hill Education; 2010.

Global Union Against Radiation Deployment from Space. "Planned Global Wi-Fi from Space Will Destroy Ozone Layer, Worsen Climate Change, and Threaten Life on Earth" [News Release], March 26, 2015. Retrieved 2018 from https://stopsmartmeters.org/global-union-against-radiation-deployment-from-space/.

Goldberg, Kim. "Sanctuaries," Refugium: Wi-Fi Exiles & The Coming Electroplague, 2015. Retrieved 2018 from https://electroplague.com/sanctuaries/.

Gonzalez, R.H. "Pesticide residues in developing countries—A review of residues detected in food exports from the developing world," *Pesticide Chemistry and Bioscience: The Food-Environment Challenge*, edited by Brooks G., and T. Roberts, Cambridge, UK: The Royal Society of Chemistry, 1999; 386–401.

Gray, Richard. "Ban mobile phones and wireless networks in schools, say European leaders," *The Telegraph*, May 14, 2011. Retrieved 2018 from https://www.telegraph.co.uk/technology/mobile-phones/8514380/Ban-mobile-phones-and-wireless-networks-in-schools-say-European-leaders.html.

Gust, Lawrence J., EE, BBEC. "Man-made Electromagnetic Radiation: What Is It and What Are the Health Effects," *Electromagnetic Radiation*, Rev 9.20.15, 1996.

Hacker Noon. "How Much Time Do People Spend on Their Mobile Phones in 2017?" May 9, 2017. Retrieved 2018 from https://hackernoon.com/how-much-time-do-people-spend-on-their-mobile-phones-in-2017-e5f90a0b10a6.

Han, S., C. Tai, R.E. Westenbroek, F.H. Yu, C.S. Cheah, G.B. Potter, J.L. Rubenstein, T. Scheuer, H.O. de la Iglesia, and W.A. Catterall. "Autistic-like behaviour in Scn1a+/- mice and rescue by enhanced GABA-mediated neurotransmission," *Nature*, September 20, 2012; 489(7416):385-90. doi: 10.1038/nature11356. Epub August 22, 2012.

Hansraj, Kenneth, MD. "Assessment of Stresses About The Cervical Spine: Caused by Posture and Position of the Head," New York Spine Surgery & Rehabilitation Medicine. Retrieved 2017 from https://realspinesurgery.com/text-neck/.

Hardell, Lennart. "A Battleground—From Phenoxyacetic Acids, Chlorophenals and Dioxins, to Mobile Phones—Cancer Risks, Greenwashing and Vested Interests," *Corporate Ties That Bind: An Examination of Corporate Manipulation and Vested Interest in Public Health*, edited by Martin J. Walker, New York, NY: Skyhorse Publishing, Inc., March 28, 2017.

Hardell, Lennart, Michael Carlberg, Kjell Hansson Mild. "Pooled analysis of two case-control studies on use of cellular and cordless telephones and the risk for malignant brain tumours diagnosed in 1997-2003," *International* Archives of *Occupational* and *Environmental Health*, March 16, 2006.

Hardell, Lennart, Tarmo Koppel, Michael Carlberg, Mikko Ahonen, and Lena Hedendahl. "Radiofrequency radiation at Stockholm Central Railway Station in Sweden and some medical aspects on public exposure to RF fields," *International Journal of Oncology*. Oct; 49(4) (2016): 1315–1324.

Hardell, L., M. Carlberg, K. Hansson Mild. "Use of Wireless Phones and Evidence for Increased risk of brain tumors," Section 11, pages 1-33. *BioInitiative 2012: A Rationale for a Biologically-based Public Exposure Standard for Electromagnetic Fields (ELF and RF),* C. Sage and D. O. Carpenter (editors). Retrieved 2017 from http://www.bioinitiative.org/.

Havas, Magda. "Austrian Medical Association guidelines for diagnosing and treating patients with electrohypersensitivity," Magdahavas.com, June 22, 2012. Retrieved 2018 from http://www.magdahavas.com/austrian-medical-association-guidelines-to-diagnosing-and-treating-patients-with-electrohypersensitivity/.

Havas, Magda. "Electromagnetic Hypersensitivity: Biological Effects of Dirty Electricity with Emphasis on Diabetes and Multiple Sclerosis," *Electromagnetic Biology and Medicine*, 25, no. 4 (2006): 259-68.

Havas, Magda. "Radiation from wireless technology affects the blood, the heart, and the autonomic nervous system," *Reviews on Environmental Health* 2013; 28(2-3): 75–84.

Hertsgaard, Mark, and Mark Dowie. "How Big Wireless Made Us Think That Cell Phones Are Safe: A Special Investigation," *The Nation*, March 29, 2018. Retrieved 2018 from https://www.thenation.com/article/how-big-wireless-made-us-think-that-cell-phones-are-safe-a-special-investigation/.

Higginbotham, Stacey. "The Future Is Now: Welcome to My (Smart) House," *Fortune*, February 17, 2017. Retrieved 2018 from http://fortune.com/2017/02/17/smart-home-tech-internet-of-things-connected-home/.

Hildenbrand, Jerry. "Does Google sell your personal data?," Android Central, Jan. 12, 2018. Retrieved January 2020 from https://www.androidcentral.com/does-google-sell-your-data.

Houlihan, Jane, Sonya Lunder, and Anila Jacob, "Timeline: BPA From Invention To Phase-Out," Environmental Working Group, April 2008 (Updated March 2011). Retrieved 2018 from https://www.ewg.org/research/timeline-bpa-invention-phase-out#.WpW3jXxG1ld.

Huber, Gary L, Robert E. Brockie, and Vijay K. Mahajan. "Passive Smoking: How Great a Hazard?" *Consumers' Research Magazine*, July, 1991.

Huber, Gary L., Robert E. Brockie, and Vijay K. Mahajan. *Passive Smoking: How Great a Hazard?*, Forest Books, 1993.

Huddleston, Brad. *Digital Cocaine: A Journey Toward iBalance* [eBook], Christian Art Publishers, 2016.

Huss, A. et al, "Source of Funding and Results of Studies of Health Effects of Mobile Phone Use: Systematic Review of Experimental Studies" *Environmental Health Perspectives*, 115, no. 1 (January 2007): 1-4.

Hyland, G.J. "Physics and biology of mobile telephony," *The Lancet*, November 25, 2000, Volume 356, No. 9244, 1833–1836.

IEEE. "Albumin leakage into the brain and wireless-communication radiation," *IEEE Antennas and Propagation Magazine*, April, 2004; 46(2),154-156.

IEMFA. "Chronic EMF-Related Diseases Are a Potential Risk for Everyone, and a Precautionary Approach Is Urgently Needed!" IEMFA Statement Stavanger, [Undated]. Retrieved 2018 from http://www.iemfa.org/iemfa-statement/.

In-cyprus.com. "Mobile devices could harm kids," December, 10, 2015. Retrieved 2018 from https://web.archive.org/web/20160131024709/http:/in-cyprus.com/mobile-devices-could-harm-kids/.

India Department of Telecom. "Ensuring Safety from Radiations: Mobile Towers and Handsets," September 1, 2012. Retrieved 2018 from www.dot.gov.in/sites/default/files/advertisement_0.pdf.

Insight Research Corp. "Worldwide Telecommunications Industry Revenue to Reach $2.4 Trillion in 2019," January 31, 2014. Retrieved 2018 from https://www.prnewswire.com/news-releases/worldwide-telecommunications-industry-revenue-to-reach-24-trillion-in-2019-says-insight-research-corp-242965161.html.

InspectAPedia. "Levels of Cancer Risk from exposure to EMF Electromagnetic Fields vs Other Cancer Risks," [Undated]. Retrieved 2018 from https://inspectapedia.com/emf/EMF_Cancer_Risk_Levels.php.

Interactive Advertising Bureau. "U.S. Firms to Spend Nearly $19.2 Billion on Third-Party Audience Data & Data-Use Solutions in 2018, Up 17.5% From 2017." Dec. 5, 2018. Retrieved January 2020 from https://www.businesswire.com/news/home/20181205005139/en/U.S.-Firms-Spend-19.2-Billion-Third-Party-Audience.

International Institute for Building-Biology & Ecology; http://hbelc.org.

International Institute for Building-Biology & Ecology. "Subtle Energy Devices: An IBE Position Paper," June 9, 2015. Retrieved 2018 from http://hbelc.org/pdf/standards/SEDs_v1.12.pdf.

Israel Environment and Health Fund and Ministry of Health. "Health in Israel 2014," 2014. Retrieved 2018 from www.health.gov.il/PublicationsFiles/BSV_sviva2014E.pdf.

Jacobo, Julia. "Teens spend more than 7 hours on screens for entertainment a day,"ABC News Special Report, October 29, 2019. Retrieved January 2020 from https://abcnews.go.com/US/teens-spend-hours-screens-entertainment-day-report/story?id=66607555.

Johansson, O. "Disturbance of the immune system by electromagnetic fields-A potentially underlying cause for cellular damage and tissue repair reduction which could lead to disease and impairment," *Pathophysiology,* 16(2-3) (August, 2009):157-77. doi: 10.1016/j.pathophys.2009.03.004.

Johansson, O., PhD. "KI-researcher: Kick out politicians who give students hazardous e-readers with unproven educational value," EMFacts Consultancy, March 14, 2014. Retrieved 2018 from https://www.emfacts.com/2014/03/is-wireless-technology-in-swedish-schools-adversely-affecting-the-kids/. Original publication: NewsVoice.se [Sweden], January 23,

2014, http://newsvoice.se/2014/01/23/ki-forskare-porta-skolpolitiker-som-vill-ge-formodat-halsofarliga-lasplattor-till-eleverna/.

Kardaras, Nicholas. *Glow Kids: How Screen Addiction Is Hijacking Our Kids—and How to Break the Trance*, Kindle Edition, New York, NY: St, Martin's Press, 2016.

Kastrenakes, Jacob. "T-Mobile to launch 5G in 30 cities this year, including New York and LA," February 27, 2018. Retrieved 2018 from https://www.theverge.com/2018/2/27/17058368/tmobile-5g-first-30-cities-2018-new-york-la-dallas-las-vegas.

Keen, Charles M. "Possible Biological Effects of Electromagnetic Fields Associated with Electric Power Systems," EMF Services, LLC, May 15, 2015. Retrieved 2018 from http://www.emfservices.com/article.htm#Epidemiology.

Kelly, Erin. "House votes to renew surveillance law that may collect Americans' emails without warrants," *USA Today*, January 11, 2018. Retrieved 2018 from https://www.usatoday.com/story/news/politics/2018/01/11/house-vote-privacy-advocates-offer-changes-controversial-surveillance/1020930001/.

Kennedy, Gail E., and Lisa A. Berob. "Print media coverage of research on passive smoking," *Tobacco Control*, 1999; 8: 254–260.

Kesari, K.K., M. Siddiqui, R. Meena, H.N. Verma, and S. Kumar. "Cell phone radiation exposure on brain and associated biological systems," *Indian Journal of Experimental Biology*, March, 2013; 188.

Khurana, Vini G., Lennart Hardell, Joris Everaert, Alicja Bortkiewicz, Michael Carlberg, and Mikko Ahonen. "Epidemiological Evidence for a Health Risk from Mobile Phone Base Stations," *International Journal of Occupational and Environmental Health*, published online: July 19, 2013; 263-267. http://www.tandfonline.com/doi/abs/10.1179/107735210799160192.

Komando, Kim. "When smart devices watch you, what do they do with the data?," *USA Today*, June 20, 2019. Retrieved January

2020 from https://www.usatoday.com/story/tech/columnist/2019/06/20/what-do-smart-devices-do-data-they-collect-you/1483051001/.

Kovarik, Bill. "The toxic history of lead," Environmental History Timeline, February 17, 2016. http://environmentalhistory.org/2016/02/17/the-toxic-history-of-lead/2016.

Kowalski, Janice, MD. "What is too much screen time doing to our kids' mental health?" Edward-Elmhurst Health, February 18, 2016. Retrieved 2018 from https://www.eehealth.org/blog/2016/02/too-much-screen-time-and-kids-mental-health/.

Kundi, M., PhD. "Evidence for Childhood Cancers (Leukemia)," BioInitiative 2012 Supplement, Rensselaer, NY: University at Albany, 2012. Retrieved 2017 from http://www.bioinitiative.org/.

Laffin, Ben, and Gina Kolata. "Will Your Cell Phone Give You Cancer?" *The New York Times*, May 27, 2016. Retrieved 2018 from https://www.nytimes.com/2016/05/28/health/cancer-study-radiation-cellphones.html

Lah, Katarina. "Effects of Pesticides on Human Health," updated May 06, 2011. Retrieved 2018 from http://www.toxipedia.org/display/toxipedia/Effects+of+Pesticides+on+Human+Health.

Lai, H. "Biological Effects of Radiofrequency Radiations," EMF—Scientific and Legal Issues, Theory and Evidence of EMF Biological and Health Effects in Catania [Symposium], Sicily, Italy, September 13-14, 2002.

Lai, H. "Evidence for Effects on Neurology and Behavior," *BioInitiative 2012: A Rationale for a Biologically-based Public Exposure Standard for Electromagnetic Fields (ELF and RF),* Section 9, August 31, 2007.

Lai, H. "Genetic Effects of Non-Ionizing Electromagnetic Fields," *BioInitiative 2012: A Rationale for a Biologically-based Public Exposure Standard for Electromagnetic Fields (ELF and RF),* Section 6 (March, 2014): 1-59. [Supplement], *BioInitiative*

2012, Rensselaer, NY: University at Albany, 2012. Retrieved 2018 from http://www.bioinitiative.org/ report/wp-content/uploads/pdfs/ sec06_2012_genetic_effects_non-ionizing.pdf.

Lai, H. "Single-and double-strand DNA breaks in rat brain cells after acute exposure to radio frequency electromagnetic radiation," *Journal of International Journal of Radiation Biology*, 69(4) (April, 1996):513-21.

Lawler, David. "From Marlboro Man to Smoking Ban: A Timeline of Tobacco in America," *The Telegraph*, November 14, 2014. Retrieved 2018 from https://www.telegraph.co.uk/ news/worldnews/northamerica/usa/11230175/From-Marlboro-Man-to-smoking-ban-a-timeline-of-tobacco-in-America.html

Lean, Geoffrey, "Mobile phone use 'raises children's risk of brain cancer fivefold,'" *Independent*, September 20, 2008. Retrieved 2018 from http://www.independent.co.uk/ news/science/mobile-phone-use-raises-childrens-risk-of-brain-cancer-fivefold-937005.html.

LeFebvre, Rob. "Hilton plans to offer a smart hotel room system next year," Engadget, Dec 7, 2017. Retrieved 2018 from https://www.engadget.com/2017/12/07/hilton-smart-hotel-room-system-next-year/.

Leong, Christopher C.W., Naweed I. Syed, and Fritz L. Lorscheider. "Mercury's Effects: Retrograde degeneration of neurite membrane structural integrity of nerve growth cones following in vitro exposure to mercury," *NeuroReport*, Volume 12, number 4 (March 26, 2001), 733-737.

Levitt, B. Blake. *Electromagnetic Fields: A Consumer's Guide to the Issues and How to Protect Ourselves,* 2nd edition. New York: Harcourt Brace, 2007.

Li, De-Kun, Hong Chen, Jeannette R. Ferber, Roxana Odouli, and Charles Quesenberry. "Exposure to Magnetic Field Non-Ionizing Radiation and the Risk of Miscarriage: A Prospective Cohort Study," *Scientific Reports*, volume 7, Article number:

17541 (2017); doi:10.1038/s41598-017-16623-8. Retrieved 2018 from https://www.nature.com/articles/ s41598-017-16623-8.

Lin, James C., and Mei F. Lin. "Microwave Hyperthermia-Induced Blood-Brain Barrier Alterations," *Radiation Research*, Vol. 89, No. 1 (January, 1982), 77-87.

Ma, Alexandra. "China has started ranking citizens with a creepy 'social credit' system—here's what you can do wrong, and the embarrassing, demeaning ways they can punish you," *Business Insider*, Oct 29, 2018. Retrieved January 2020 https://www.businessinsider.com/china-social-credit-system-punishments-and-rewards-explained-2018-4.

Macdonald, Cheyenne. "Bizarre babypod 'tampon speaker' can play music to unborn children," *Daily Mail*, January 5, 2016. Retrieved 2018 from http://www.dailymail.co.uk/sciencetech/article-3386181/Bizarre-babypod-tampon-speaker-play-music-unborn-children.html#ixzz5ADLGH2w8.

Margalit, Liraz, PhD. "What Screen Time Can Really Do to Kids' Brains: Too much at the worst possible age can have lifetime consequences," *Psychology Today*, April 17, 2016. Retrieved 2018 from https://www.psychologytoday.com/us/comment/856244.

Mariea, Tamara. "Research on Correlation Between Autism, Cell Phones, and Wireless Computers" [News Release], Internal Balance, April 16, 2007. Retrieved 2018 from businesswire.com/news/home/20070416006297/en/Research-Correlation-Autism-Cell-Phones-Wireless-Computers.

Mariea, Tamara, and G.L. Carlo, "Wireless Radiation in the Etiology and Treatment of Autism: Clinical Observations and Mechanisms," *Journal of the Australasian College of Nutritional and Environmental Medicine*, 26, no. 2, 2007.

Marino, A.A. "Are powerline fields hazardous to health?" *Public Power*, 1987, 45:1820.

Marino, A.A., and D.M. Morris. "Chronic electromagnetic stressors in the environment: A risk factor in human cancer," A.A. Marino & D.M. Morris. *Journal of Environmental Science*, 1985, C3(2):189–219.

Marino, A.A. "Electromagnetic energy in the environment and human disease," *Clinical Ecology*, 1985, 3(3):154–157.

Marino, A.A. "Electromagnetic fields and public health," *Assessments and Viewpoints on the Biological and Human Health Effects of Extremely Low Frequency Electromagnetic Fields*, American Institute of Biological Sciences, Arlington, Va., 1985, 205–232.

Marino, A.A. "Electromagnetic fields, cancer, and the theory of neuroendocrine-related promotion," *Journal of Bioelectrochemistry and Bioenergetics*, 1993; 29:255–276.

Marino, A.A. "Environmental electromagnetic fields and public health," *Foundations of Modern Bioelectricity*, ed. Marcel Dekker, New York: CRC Press, 1988, 965–1044.

Marino, A.A. "Health risks from electric power facilities," *Proceedings of International Utility Symposium, Health Effects of Electric and Magnetic Fields*, Ontario Hydro, Toronto, 1986.

Marr, Bernard. "Chinese Social Credit Score: Utopian Big Data Bliss Or Black Mirror On Steroids?," *Forbes*, Jan. 21, 2019. Retrieved January 2020 from https://www.forbes.com/sites/bernardmarr/2019/01/21/chinese-social-credit-score-utopian-big-data-bliss-or-black-mirror-on-steroids/#325c8bc848b8.

Mathias, Craig. "A brief-history-of-wireless-technology," *IT World*, March 22, 2004. Retrieved 2018 from itworld.com/article/2802953/mobile/a-brief-history-of-wireless-technology.html.

Mazar, H. "A Global Survey and Comparison of Different Regulatory Approaches to Non-Ionizing RADHAZ and Spurious Emissions," Ministry of Communications, RF Spectrum Department, Israel, November 9, 2009.

Mearian, Lucas. "Wireless charging explained: What is it and how does it work?" *Computer World*, October 31, 2017. Retrieved 2018 from https://www.computerworld.com/article/3235176/mobile-wireless/wireless-charging-explained-what-is-it-and-how-does-it-work.html.

MediaPost. "Google Search Chip Inside The Brain, A," October 25, 2010. Retrieved 2018 from mediapost.com/publications/article/138263/a-google-search-chip-inside-the-brain.html.

Media Tech Reviews. “The number of cell phone users in the United States in 2018 amounted to 237.72 million,” March 20, 2018. Retrieved 2018 from mediatechreviews.com/how-many-cell-phone-subscribers-the-us/.

Mercola, Joseph, DO. “Cell Phone Gave Man a Tumor, According to Major Court Ruling,” November 07, 2012. Retrieved 2018 from https://articles.mercola.com/sites/articles/archive/2012/11/07/heavy-cell-phone-use.aspx.

Mercola, Joseph, DO. “Dr. Mercola Interviews Martin Pall on EMFs” [Video], Mercola YouTube channel, Aug 30, 2017. Retrieved 2018 from youtube.com/watch?v=ZAqmT9KJBC8.

Mercola, Joseph, DO. “EMF Controversy Exposed.” January 20, 2016. Retrieved 2018 from https://articles.mercola.com/sites/articles/archive/2016/01/20/emf-controversy-exposed.aspx.

Mercola, Joseph, DO. “European Union Bans Amalgam Fillings for Children and Pregnant or Nursing Women,” Wake Up World. Retrieved 2018 from https://wakeup-world.com/2017/01/18/european-union-bans-amalgam-fillings-for-children-and-pregnant-or-nursing-women/.

Mercola, Joseph, DO. “The Harmful Effects of Electromagnetic Fields Explained,” Wake Up World, December 22, 2017. Retrieved 2018 from https://wakeup-world.com/2017/12/22/the-harmful-effects-of-electromagnetic-fields-explained/.

Mercola, Joseph, DO. “Yet Another Reason Not to Hold Your Cellphone,” Mercola: Take Control of Your Health, September 09, 2017. Retrieved 2018 from https://articles.mercola.com/sites/articles/archive/2017/09/09/cellphone-usage-health-risks.aspx.

Mesotheliona.guide. “Asbestos and the Law: Future Civil Litigation.” Retrieved 2018 from mesothelioma.guide/lawsuits/future-litigation.html.

MesotheliomaHelp. “Asbestos Timeline,” [Undated]. Retrieved 2018 from https://www.mesotheliomahelp.org/asbestos/history/.

Meyer, David. "Vladimir Putin Says Whoever Leads in Artificial Intelligence Will Rule the World," *Fortune*, September 4, 2017. Retrieved January 2020 from https://fortune.com/2017/09/04/ai-artificial-intelligence-putin-rule-world/.

Microwave News. "Power-Frequency EMFs Promote Cancer in Massive Animal Study: Italians Call for a 'Reevaluation of the Safety of Non-Ionizing Radiation,'" February 27, 2016. Retrieved 2018 from http://microwavenews.com/news-center/ramazzini-animal-study.

Microwave News. "What Changed at NTP? Same RF Cancer Data, Different Outlook," February 7, 2018. Retrieved 2018 from http://microwavenews.com/news-center/what-changed.

Milham. Dr. Samuel. *Dirty Electricity—Electrification and the Diseases of Civilization*, 2nd Edition, iUniverse, 2012.

Miller, Chance. "Ahead of CES, Apple touts 'what happens on your iPhone, stays on your iPhone' with privacy billboard in Las Vegas," 9to5Mac, Jan. 5, 2019. https://9to5mac.com/2019/01/05/apple-privacy-billboard-vegas-ces/.

Miller, Lawrence. *5G RF for Dummies*, Quorvo Special Edition, Hoboken, NJ: John Wiley & Sons, Inc., 2017.

Miller, Lawrence. *Internet of Things Applications for Dummies*, Hoboken, NJ: John Wiley & Sons, Inc., 2017.

Milner, Conan. "The Dark Side of Wireless Technology," *Epoch Times*, January 17, 2018. Retrieved 2018 from www.theepochtimes.com/the-dark-side-of-wireless-technology_2403062.html.

Mihai, Teodor, Pincu Rotinberg, Florin Brinza, and Gabriela Vochita. "Extremely low-frequency electromagnetic fields cause DNA strand breaks in normal cells," *Journal of Environmental Health Science & Engineering*, published online January 8, 2014; 12: 15. doi: 10.1186/2052-336X-12-15.

Mole, Beth. "California: Here's how to handle unfounded fears of cell phone cancer," Ars Technica, December 16, 2017. Retrieved 2018 from arstechnica.com/science/ 2017/ 12/california-heres-how-to-handle-unfounded-fears-of-cell-phone-cancer/.

Monroe Toxicology. "Timeline on the Toxicology of Lead," HG.org Legal Resources, [Undated]. Retrieved 2018 from https://www.hg.org/article.asp?id=21970.

Morgan, Lloyd. "Excess Risk of Brain Cancer with 5 Years or More, and/or Cellphone Use on Same Side of Head as Tumor Location or, Combinations of Wireless Phone Use: Interphone Results Versus Swedish Team Results," Power Watch, August, 18, 2006. Retrieved 2018 from powerwatch.org.uk/columns/morgan/20060818_viewgraphs.asp.

Morgan, Lloyd. "The Latest Study on the Risk of Brain Cancer From Wireless Phone Use," Power Watch, August 17, 2006. Retrieved 2018 from http://powerwatch.org.uk/columns/morgan/20060817_wireless_tumours.asp?pf=1.

Morgan, Lloyd. "Scientists manipulated research on brain tumour risk for children (Part 1)," EMFacts Consultancy, Oct 2, 2011. Retrieved 2018 from https://www.emfacts.com/2011/10/scientists-manipulated-research-on-brain-tumour-risk-for-children-part-1/.

Moskowitz, Joel M., PhD. "5G Wireless Technology: Millimeter Wave Health Effects" [Blog], Electromagnetic Radiation Safety, August 7, 2017. Retrieved 2018 from saferemr.com/2017/08/5g-wireless-technology-millimeter-wave.html.

Moskowitz, Joel M., PhD. "The European Commission responds with denial and empty promises to scientists and doctors demanding a moratorium on 5G" [Blog], Electromagnetic Radiation Safety, October 25, 2017. Retrieved 2018 from http://www.saferemr.com/2017/09/5G-moratorium12.html.

Moskowitz, Joel M., PhD. "National Toxicology Program (NTP) Cell Phone Radiation 2-Year Study—Evaluation of Carcinogenicity of Cell Phone Radiation: NTP Draft Technical Reports (TR 595, TR 596) vs. Expert Panel Vote," School of Public Health, UC Berkeley, March 28, 2018. Retrieved 2018 from http://www.emfsa.co.za/wp-content/uploads/2018/03/180328_summary-of-NTP-expert-panel-recommendations.pdf.

Mother Jones. "The Tobacco Wars," May/June 1996. Retrieved 2018 from http://www.motherjones.com/politics/1996/05/tobacco-wars-6/.

National Archives (U.S.). "The Kite Experiment, October 19, 1752," [Undated]. Retrieved 2018 from founders.archives.gov/documents/Franklin/01-04-02-0135.

National Cancer Institute. "Cell Phones and Cancer Risk" [Fact Sheet], [Undated]. Retrieved 2018 from https://www.cancer.gov/ about-cancer/causes-prevention/risk/radiation/cell-phones-fact-sheet.

National Cancer Institute. "Formaldehyde and Cancer Risk," [Undated]. Retrieved 2018 from https://www.cancer.gov/about-cancer/causes-prevention/risk/substances/formaldehyde/formaldehyde-fact-sheet.

National Research Council. "Table 10-2: General Public Exposure Standards or Guidelines for Several Countries or Agencies," *Assessment of the Possible Health Effects of Ground Wave Emergency Network, National Research Council (U.S.) Committee on Assessment of the Possible Health Effects of Ground Wave Emergency Network (GWEN)*, Washington, DC: National Academies Press, 1993.

Natural Society. "Radiation: Unsafe at Any Dose," [Undated]. Retrieved 2017 from http://naturalsociety.com/radiation-unsafe-at-any-dose/#ixzz5803s9NKo.

Naydler, Jeremy, PhD. "5G – The Big Picture," Take Back Your Power, April 2019. Retrieved January 2020 from https://takebackyourpower.net/5g-the-big-picture/.

Nelson, Patrick. "We touch our phones 2,617 times a day, says study," Network World, July 7, 2016. Retrieved 2018 from https://www.networkworld.com/article/3092446/smartphones/we-touch-our-phones-2617-times-a-day-says-study.html.

New England Journal of Medicine. "Dioxin Controversy," [Undated]. Retrieved 2018 from https://www.uow.edu.au/~sharonb/STS218/dioxin/pr/journal.html.

Nittby, H., G. Grafstrom, D.P. Tian. "Cognitive impairment in rats after long-term exposure to GSM-900 mobile phone radiation," *Bioelectromagnetics*, April, 2008; 29(3): 219-32.

No Radiation For You [blog]; http://www.norad4u.com.

Nyberg, Rainer, and Lennart Hardell et al. "5G Appeal: Scientists and doctors warn of potential serious health effects of 5G," Scientists Appeal for 5G Moratorium, September 13, 2017. Retrieved 2018 from iemfa.org/news/scientists-and-doctors-appeal-for-5g-moratorium-warn-of-potential-serious-health-effects-of-5g/.

Olson, David A., MD. "Mercury Toxicity," Medscape, updated: Aug 14, 2017. Retrieved 2017 from https://emedicine.medscape.com/article/1175560-overview.

Oscar, K.J., and T.D. Hawkins. "Microwave Alteration of the Blood-Brain Barrier System of Rats," *Brain Research*, Vol. 126 (1977), 281-293.

Oxford Dictionaries; https://en.oxforddictionaries.com.

Paknahad, Maryam, et al. "Effect of radiofrequency radiation from Wi-Fi devices on mercury release from amalgam restorations," *Journal of Environmental Health Science Engineering*, July 13, 2016. Published online July 13, 2016 . doi: 10.1186/s40201-016-0253-z. Retrieved 2018 from https://www.ncbi.nlm.nih.gov/pmc/articles/PMC4944481/.

Pallister, James. "Will the Internet of Things set family life back 100 years?" Medium.com, September 3, 2015. Retrieved 2018 from https://medium.com/@DesignCouncil/will-the-internet-of-things-set-family-life-back-100-years-18ce46b96646.

Parents for Safe Technology; parentsforsafetechnology.org.

Parents For Safe Technology. "Worldwide Precautionary Action," [Undated]. Retrieved 2018 from http://www.parentsforsafetechnology.org/worldwide-countries-taking-action.html.

Patel, Prachi. "Wireless Phone Charging Picks Up Steam," *Scientific American*, March 3, 2017. Retrieved 2018 from https://www.scientificamerican.com/article/wireless-phone-charging-picks-up-steam/.

Paul, Kari. "'Smart' hotel rooms will know how you like to sleep," *New York Post*, Oct 2, 2017. Retrieved 2018 from https://nypost.com/2017/10/02/smart-hotel-rooms-will-know-how-you-like-to-sleep/.

Paz de la Puente, Maria, and Alfonso Balmori. "Addiction to cell phones. Are there neurophysiological mechanisms involved?" Proyecto de ley 61, Panama, March, 2007. Abstract retrieved 2017 from https://www.researchgate.net/publication/238032691_Addiction_to_cell_phones_Are_there_neurophysiological_mechanisms_involved.

PBS. "Internet Addiction around the World," February 2, 2010. Retrieved 2018 from https://www.pbs.org/wgbh/pages/frontline/digitalnation/virtual-worlds/internet-addiction/internet-rescue-camp.html.

PBS Frontline. "Timeline: Endocrine Disruption and Man-made Chemicals," [Undated]. Retrieved 2018 from www.pbs.org/wgbh/pages/frontline/shows/nature/etc/cron.html.

Pesticide Action Network. "The DDT Story," May 29, 2009. Retrieved 2018 from www.panna.org/resources/ddt-story.

PetFinder.com. "How Do Pet Microchips Work?" [Undated]. Retrieved 2018 from https://www.petfinder.com/dogs/lost-and-found-dogs/how-pet-microchips-work/.

Pew Research Center. "Mobile Fact Sheet," February 5, 2018. Retrieved 2018 from pewinternet.org/fact-sheet/mobile/.

Pineault, Nicolas. *The Non-Tinfoil Guide to EMFs: How to Fix Our Stupid Use of Technology*, N&G Média, Inc., 2017, 143.

Plourde, Elizabeth, PhD, and Marcus Plourde, PhD. *EMF Freedom, Solutions for the 21st Century Pollution*, 3rd Edition, Irvine, CA: New Voice Publications, 2016.

Pollack, Andrew. "Questions and Answers on the New Study Linking Cellphones and Cancer in Rats," *The New York Times*, May 27, 2016. Retrieved 2018 from https://www.nytimes.com/2016/05/28/health/cancer-study-radiation-cellphones.html.

Portier, C., A. Tritscher, M. Kohn, C. Sewall, G. Clark, L. Edler, D. Hoel and G. Lucier. "Ligand/Receptor Binding for 2,3,7,8-

TCDD: Implications for Risk Assessment," *Toxicological Sciences*, Volume 20, Issue 1, January 1, 1993, 48-56, https://doi.org/10.1093/toxsci/20.1.48.

Prasad, M., P. Kathuria, P. Nair, A. Kumar, K. Prasad. "Mobile phone use and risk of brain tumours: a systematic review of association between study quality, source of funding, and research outcomes," *Journal of the Neurological Sciences*, 2017; 38 (5): 797-810; doi:10.1007/s10072-017-2850-8.

Preece, A.W., J.W. Hand, R.N. Clarke, and A. Stewart. "Power frequency electromagnetic fields and health. Where's the evidence?," *Physics in Medicine & Biology*, September 2000; 45(9): R139-54.

Priest, David. "Smart homes might be getting too smart. Start worrying. Commentary: When better features mean worse ethics, should we change what we buy?," CNET, October 31, 2019. Retrieved January 2020 from https://www.cnet.com/news/smart-homes-might-be-getting-too-smart-start-worrying/.

Proctor, Robert N. *The Nazi War on Cancer*, Princeton, NJ: Princeton University Press, 1999.

Proctor, Robert N. "The shameful past: The history of the discovery of the cigarette–lung cancer link: evidentiary traditions, corporate denial, global toll," Tobacco Control, 16 February, 2012. Retrieved 2018 from http://tobaccocontrol.bmj.com/content/21/2/87.

Prospero, Mike. "Best Smart Home Gadgets of 2018," Tom's Guide, February 26, 2018. Retrieved 2018 from https://www.tomsguide.com/us/best-smart-home-gadgets,review-2008.html.

Purcell, Edward M., and David J. Morin. *Electricity and Magnetism.* New York, NY: Cambridge University Press, 2013.

Radiant Insights, Inc. "U.S. Telecom Market Size to Reach $1.3 Trillion by 2020" [News Release], March 30, 2016. Retrieved 2018 from http://www.marketwired.com/press-release/us-telecom-market-size-to-reach-13-trillion-by-2020-radiant-insights-inc-2110041.htm.

Rainie, Lee. "Cell phone ownership hits 91% of adults," Pew Research Center, June 6, 2013. Retrieved 2018 from http://www.pewresearch.org/fact-tank/2013/06/06/cell-phone-ownership-hits-91-ofadults/.
Reardon, Marguerite. "The trouble with the cell phone radiation standard: The standard used by federal regulators may not be the best measure of safety, nor is it the best way to help concerned consumers reduce their exposure," *CNET Magazine*, June 2, 2011. Retrieved 2018 from https://www.cnet.com/news/the-trouble-with-the-cell-phone-radiation-standard/.
Redmayne, M. "International policy and advisory response regarding children's exposure to radio frequency electromagnetic fields, (RF-EMF)," *Electromagnetic Biology* and *Medicine*, 2016; 35(2):176-85. doi: 10.3109/ 15368378.2015.1038832.
Reichert, Corinne. "AT&T 5G coming to Dallas, Atlanta, Waco in 2018," CNET, February 21, 2018. Retrieved 2018 from http://www.zdnet.com/article/at-t-5g-coming-to-dallas-atlanta-waco-in-2018/.
Reinhardt, Claudia, and Bill Ganzel. "Farming in the 1930s: DDT," Wessels Living History Farm, 2003. Retrieved 2018 from livinghistoryfarm.org/farminginthe30s/pests_05.html.
Reinhardt, Claudia, and Bill Ganzel. "Farming in the 1940s: Insecticides – DDT +," Wessels Living History Farm, 2003. Retrieved 2018 from https://livinghistoryfarm.org/farminginthe40s/pests_02.html.
Robertson, Sally, BSc. "Lead Poisoning History," *News Medical & Life Sciences*, [Undated]. Retrieved 2018 from www.news-medical.net/health/Lead-Poisoning-History.aspx.
Rosenbaum, Eric. "Tech spending will near $4 trillion this year. Here's where all the money is going and why," CNBC, April 8, 2019. Retrieved January 2020 from https://www.cnbc.com/2019/04/08/4-trillion-in-tech-spending-in-2019-heres-where-the-money-is-going.html.
Ruff, Kathleen. "Serving Industry, Promoting Skepticism, Discrediting Epidemiology," *Corporate Ties That Bind: An*

Examination of Corporate Manipulation and Vested Interest in Public Health, edited by Martin J. Walker, New York, NY: Skyhorse Publishing, Inc., Mar 28, 2017.

Russian National Committee of Non-Ionizing Radiation Protection. "Russian National Committee of Non-Ionizing Radiation Protection, 2008 report," 2008. Retrieved 2018 from http://www.who.int/peh-emf/project/mapnatreps/RUSSIA%20report%202008.pdf.

Safe Living Technologies, Inc. "EMR Exposure Guidelines," [Undated]. Retrieved 2018 from slt.co/Education/EMR-ExposureGuidelines.aspx.

SafeSpace. "Is Cell Tower Radiation Dangerous?" [Undated]. Retrieved 2018 from https://www.safespaceprotection.com/emf-health-risks/emf-health-effects/cell-towers/.

Sage, C. (ed.). *BioInitiative 2007—A Rationale for a Biologically-based Public Exposure Standard for Electromagnetic Fields (ELF and RF),* Rensselaer, NY: University at Albany, 2007. Retrieved 2017 from http://www.bioinitiative.org/.

Sage, C. (ed.). "Conclusions – Table 1-1" *BioInitiative 2012—A Rationale for a Biologically-based Public Exposure Standard for Electromagnetic Fields (ELF and RF),* BioInitiative Report, Rensselaer, NY: University at Albany, 2012, [Genetics and Neurological Effects updated March 2014]. Retrieved 2018 from bioinitiative.org/ report/wp-content/uploads/pdfs/section_1_table_1_ 2012.pdf.

Saint, Nick. "Eric Schmidt: Google's Policy Is To 'Get Right Up To The Creepy Line And Not Cross It,'" *Business Insider*, October 1, 2010. Retrieved 2018 from http://www.businessinsider.com/eric-schmidt-googles-policy-is-to-get-right-up-to-the-creepy-line-and-not-cross-it-2010-10.

Salford, L.G., H. Nittby, and B.R.R. Persson. "Effects of Electromagnetic Fields From Wireless Communication upon the Blood-Brain Barrier," *BioInitiative 2012: A Rationale for a Biologically-based Public Exposure Standard for Electromagnetic Fields (ELF and RF),* Section 10. BioInitiative

Report, Rensselaer, NY: University at Albany, 2012. Retrieved 2017 from http://www.bioinitiative.org/.

Santini, R., P. Santini, P. Le Ruz, J.M. Danze, and M. Seignel. "Survey Study of People Living in the Vicinity of Cellular Phone Base Stations," *Electronicmagnetic Biology and Medicine* (2003) Vol. 22, No. 1, 4149.

Sapien, Joaquin. "A Timeline of CDC's and FEMA's Response to Formaldehyde Danger," ProPublica, October 5, 2008. Retrieved 2018 from https://www.propublica.org/article/formaldehyde-document-timeline.

Sara. "EMF Quiet Zones," EMFs.com, January 19, 2014. Retrieved 2018 from http://www.emfs.com/article/emf-quiet-zones.

Savitz, D.A., H. Wachtel, F.A. Barnes, E.M. John, and J.G. Tvrdik. "Case-control study of childhood cancer and exposure to 60-Hz magnetic fields," *American Journal of Epidemiology* 1988; 128:21-38.

Savitz, D.A., and E.E. Calle. "Leukemia and occupational exposure to electromagnetic fields," Review of epidemiologic surveys, *Journal of Occupational Medicine*, 1987; 29:47-51.

Savitz, D.A., N.E. Pearce, and C. Poole. "Methodological issues in the epidemiology of electromagnetic fields and cancer," *Epidemiologic Reviews*, 1989; 11:59-78.

Schumaker, Erin. "10 Statistics that Capture the Dangers of Texting and Driving," *Huffington Post*, July 7, 2015. Retrieved 2018 from https://www.huffingtonpost.com/ 2015/06/08/dangers-of-texting-and-driving-statistics_n_7537710.html.

Sedona Smart Meter Awareness [Facebook Group]. Retrieved 2018 from facebook.com/SedonaSmartMeterAwareness/.

Senum, Reinette. "The 5G Network: What you don't know may kill you," *Nexus Magazine*, April 2017. Retrieved 2017 from https://www.scribd.com/document/361776193/5G-What-You-Don-t-Know-May-Kill-You.

Shapiro, Robert, and Siddhartha Aneja. "Who Owns Americans' Personal Information and What Is It Worth?," Future Majority, March 8, 2019. Retrieved January 2020 from https://assets.futuremajority.org/uploads/report-for-future-majority-on-the-value-of-people-s-personal-data-shapiro-aneja-march-8-2019.pdf.

Siat, Sven. "Back to the Future. The State of Hotel Room Technology," Medium.com, Jan 19, 2017. Retrieved 2018 from https://medium.com/spark-innovation/back-to-the-future-the-state-of-hotel-room-technology-abcdcfd7061.

Singer, Katie. *An Electronic Silent Spring*, Great Barrington, MA: Portal Books, 2014.

Singh, Sarika, and Neeru Kapoor. "Health Implications of Electromagnetic Fields, Mechanisms of Action, and Research Needs," *Advances in Biology*, Volume 2014 (2014), Article ID 198609, 24 pages. Retrieved 2018 from http://dx.doi.org/10.1155/2014/198609.

Slesin, Louis, PhD (editor & publisher). "'More Than a Coincidence': New Large Animal Study, Like NTP's, Links RF to Schwannoma of the Heart," *Microwave News*, February 20, 2018; updated March 6, 2018. Retrieved 2018 from http://microwavenews.com/news-center/more-coincidence.

Slesin, Louis, PhD (editor & publisher). "Power-Frequency EMFs Promote Cancer in Massive Animal Study: Italians Call for a 'Reevaluation of the Safety of Non-Ionizing Radiation.' " *Microwave News: A Report on Non-Ionizing Radiation*, May 24, 2016. Retrieved 2018 from http://microwavenews.com/ news-center/ramazzini-animal-study.

Sloane, Julie. "Mercury: Element of the Ancients," Dartmouth Toxic Metals Superfund Research Program. Retrieved 2017 from www.dartmouth.edu/~toxmetal/mercury/history.html.

Snowden, Edward. "How Your Cell Phone Spies on You," YouTube, Oct. 23, 2019. Retrieved January 2020 from https://www.youtube.com/watch?v=VFns39RXPrU.

Sol, Josh del (director). *Take Back Your Power* [Documentary Film]. USA, 2017.

Statistics Portal. "Global revenue from telecommunications services from 2005 to 2019," [Undated]. Retrieved 2018 from https://www.statista.com/statistics/268628/ worldwide-revenue-from-telecommunications-services-since-2005/.

Statistics Portal. "Revenue of major U.S. wireless telecommunication providers in 2016," [Undated] . Retrieved 2018 from www.statista.com/statistics/ 201048/total-operating-revenues-of-us-telecommunication-providers/Stepansky, R., et al. "Electromagnetic fields—effects on health," Acta Med Austriaca, 2000.

Stern, Joanna. "Smart Tampon? The Internet of Every Single Thing Must Be Stopped," *Wall Street Journal*, May 25, 2016. Retrieved 2018 from https://www.wsj.com/articles/smart-tampon-the-internet-of-every-single-thing-must-be-stopped-1464198157.

Stewart, Sir William. "Evidence of a Cell Phone Risk Stronger Today than in 2000," BBC, November 20, 2006. Retrieved 2018 from http://news.bbc.co.uk/2/hi/health/4163003.stm.

Stillman, Jessica. "Why Steve Jobs and Bill Gates Both Severely Limited Their Kids' Tech Use: They built our tech-obsessed world, but they wanted something different for their own kids,", Inc.com, October 29, 2017. Retrieved 2018 from https://www.inc.com/jessica-stillman/why-steve-jobs-bill-gates-both-severely-limited-their-kids-tech-use.html.

Sutori.com. "Tobacco Timeline," [Undated]. Retrieved 2018 from https://www.sutori.com/story/tobacco-timeline-6bc8.

Szal, Andy. "California Governor Vetoes Statewide 5G Antenna Standards," *Wireless Week*, October 16, 2017. Retrieved 2018 from https://www.wirelessweek.com/news/2017/10/ california-governor-vetoes-statewide-5g-antenna-standards.

Szal, Andy. "Trump Administration Includes 5G in National Security Outline," *Wireless Week*, December 12, 2017. Retrieved 2018 from wirelessweek.com/news/2017/12/ trump-administration-includes-5g-national-security-outline.

Taylor, C. Barr, MD, and Joel D. Killen, PhD. *The Facts About Smoking*, Yonkers, NY: Consumer Reports Books, 1992.

Tang J, Y. Zhang, L. Yang L et al. "Exposure to 900 MHz electromagnetic fields activates the mkp-1/ERK pathway and causes blood-brain barrier damage and cognitive impairment in rats," *Brain Research*, March 19. 2015; 1601:92-101. doi: 10.1016/j.brainres.2015.01.019. Epub, January 15, 2015.

Thompson, Stuart A., and Charlie Warzel. "One Nation, Tracked An Investigation into the Smartphone Tracking Industry," *The New York Times*, Dec. 19, 2019. Retrieved January 2020 from https://www.nytimes.com/interactive/2019/12/19/opinion/location-tracking-cell-phone.html.

TheVerge.com. "Exclusive: Intel's new smart glasses hands-on," Feb 5, 2018. Retrieved 2018 from youtu.be/bnfwClgheFo.

Thornton, I.M. "Out of Time: A Possible Link between Mirror Neurons, Autism and Electromagnetic Radiation," *Medical Hypotheses*, 2006; 67(2):378-82. Epub March 10, 2006.

Titan Environmental. "Timeline of Lead, A, " September 2013. Retrieved 2018 from https://www.titankc.com/a-timeline-of-lead/.Tobacco Industry Research Committee. "A Frank Statement to Cigarette Smokers" [Advertisement], January 4, 1954. Retrieved 2018 from http://archive.tobacco.org/Documents/dd/ddfrankstatement.html.

Tobacco Institute. "Smoking and Health: The Need to Know [Parts 1-2]," [Documentary Film], 1972.

Toh, Michelle. "5G is helping make Pyeongchang the most high-tech Olympics ever," CNN, February 19, 2018. Retrieved 2018 from http://money.cnn.com/2018/02/19/technology/pyeongchang-winter-olympics-5g-intel/index.html.

Townsend, Peter. *The Dark Side of Technology*, Oxford, England: Oxford University Press, 1st edition, March 12, 2017.

Tran, Minh, DMD. "Accurate Location Accurate Location Detection," Federal Communications Commission, May 6, 2015. Retrieved January 2020 from https://transition.fcc.gov/pshs/911/Apps%20Wrkshp%202015/911_Help_SMS_WhitePaper0515.pdf.

Trump, Donald. "National Security Strategy of the United States of America," The White House, December 19, 2017. Retrieved 2018 from https://www.whitehouse.gov/wp-content/uploads/2017/12/NSS-Final-12-18-2017-0905.pdf.

Turner, Ash. "How Many Smartphones Are in the World? January 2020 Mobile User Statistics," BankMyCell, [Undated]. Retrieved Feb. 19, 2020, from https://www.bankmycell.com/blog/how-many-phones-are-in-the-world.

Tweedale, Geoffrey. "Secret Ties in Asbestos—Downplaying and Effacing the Risks of a Toxic Mineral," *Corporate Ties That Bind: An Examination of Corporate Manipulation and Vested Interest in Public Health*, edited by Martin J. Walker, New York, NY: Skyhorse Publishing, Inc., March 28, 2017.

Union of Concerned Scientists. "How Fossil Fuel Lobbyists Used 'Astroturf' Front Groups to Confuse the Public," Center for Science and Democracy. Retrieved 2018 from https://www.ucsusa.org/using-astroturf-front-groups-hide-fossil-fuel-lobbying-efforts#.WpW8y3xG1lc.

U.S. Department of Health and Human Services, National Toxicology Program. "Cell Phones: The draft NTP Technical Reports on rats and mice will undergo peer review by an external expert panel March 26-28, 2018," [Undated]. Retrieved 2018 from https://ntp.niehs.nih.gov/results/areas/ cellphones/.

U.S. Department of Health and Human Services, National Toxicology Program. "NTP Technical Report on the Toxicology and Carcinogenesis Studies in B6c3f1/N Mice Exposed to Whole-Body Radio Frequency Radiation at a Frequency (1,900 Mhz) and Modulations (GSM and CDMA) Used by Cell Phones," [Abstract for TR-596], February 2018. Retrieved 2018 from https://ntp.niehs.nih.gov/go/tr596abs.

U.S. Department of Health and Human Services, National Toxicology Program. "Report of Partial findings from the National Toxicology Program Carcinogenesis Studies of Cell Phone Radiofrequency Radiation in Hsd: Sprague Dawley SD

rats (Whole Body Exposure)," May 26, 2016. Retrieved 2018 from https://doi.org/10.1101/055699.
U.S. Department of Health and Human Services, National Toxicology Program. "Telephone Press Conference: NTP Draft Conclusions for Radiofrequency Radiation Studies in Rats and Mice," Feb. 2, 2018. Retrieved 2018 from niehs.nih.gov/news/newsroom/releases/2018/february2/radiofrequency_508.pdf.
U.S. Environmental Protection Agency. "Compact Fluorescent Light Bulbs (CFLs)," [Undated]. Retrieved 2018 from https://www.epa.gov/cfl.
U.S. Environmental Protection Agency. "Environmental Assessment—Dioxin," 2003. Retrieved 2018 from https://semspub.epa.gov/work/01/505090.pdf.
U.S. Environmental Protection Agency. "Health Assessment Document for Polychlorinated Dibenzo-P-Dioxins" [Abstract], Washington, DC, EPA/600/8-84/014F (NTIS PB86122546), 1985. Retrieved 2018 from cfpub.epa.gov/ncea/risk/recordisplay.cfm?deid=38484.
U.S. Food & Drug Administration. "Bisphenol A (BPA): Use in Food Contact Application; Update on Bisphenol A (BPA) for Use in Food Contact Applications," updated November 2014. Retrieved 2018 from https://www.fda.gov/newsevents/publichealthfocus/ucm064437.htm.
U.S. House of Representatives. "Toxic Trailers—Toxic Lethargy: How the Centers for Disease Control and Prevention has Failed to Protect the Public Health," Majority Staff Report Subcommittee on Investigations & Oversight Committee on Science & Technology, September, 2008.
Van Strum, Carol, and Paul E. Merrell. *No margin of safety: a preliminary report on dioxin pollution and the need for emergency action in the pulp and paper industry*. Toronto, Ontario: Greenpeace, USA, Inc., 1987.
Villas-Boas, Antonio, and Jeff Dunn. "Our Wireless Future: All the tech that's available today, and what's coming in the next 10

years," *Business Insider*, October 13, 2016. Retrieved 2018 from https://businessinsider.com/wireless-tech-2016-9.

Vogel, Sarah A., PhD, MPH, MEM. "The Politics of Plastics: The Making and Unmaking of Bisphenol A 'Safety'" *American Journal of Public Health*, November 2009; 99(Suppl 3): S559–S566. doi: 10.2105/AJPH.2008.159228.

Volkow, N.D., et al. "Effects of cell phone radiofrequency signal exposure on brain glucose metabolism," *JAMA*, Feb 23, 2011; 305(8): 808-13. doi: 10.1001/jama.2011.186.

Walleczek, J. "Electromagnetic field effects on cells of the immune system: the role of calcium signaling," *FASEB Journal*, 6(13) (October, 1992):3177-85.

Wamsley, Laurel. "France Moves To Ban Students From Using Cellphones In Schools," NPR, December 12, 2017. Retrieved 2018 from https://www.npr.org/sections/thetwo-way/2017/12/ 12/570145408/france-moves-to-ban-students-from-using-cellphones-in-schools.

Waseem, Mohammed. "A smart wallet that will be very, very hard to lose," *The Times of India*, Jul 20, 2017. Retrieved 2018 from https://timesofindia.indiatimes.com/city/ bengaluru/a-smart-wallet-that-will-be-very-very-hard-to-lose/articleshow/59664284.cms.

Weinschenk, Susan, PhD. "Why We're All Addicted to Texts, Twitter and Google, " *Psychology Today*, September 11, 2012. Retrieved 2017 from www.psychologytoday.com/ blog/brain-wise/201209/why-were-all-addicted-texts-twitter-and-google.

Weisskopf, Michael. "Paper Industry Campaign Defused Reaction to Dioxin Contamination," *Washington Post*, October 25, 1987. Retrieved 2018 from https://www.washingtonpost.com/archive/politics/1987/10/25/paper-industry-campaign-defused-reaction-to-dioxin-contamination/e95770b0-160b-4efd-b0b6-730648245c86/.

Weller, Chris. "Bill Gates and Steve Jobs raised their kids tech-free—and it should've been a red flag," *Business Insider*, January 10, 2018. Retrieved 2018 from

http://www.businessinsider.com/screen-time-limits-bill-gates-steve-jobs-red-flag-2017-10.
Wertheimer, N., and E. Leeper. "Electrical Wiring Configurations and Childhood Cancer," *American Journal of Epidemiology*, March 1979, 109(3):273-84.
White, Larry C. *Merchants of Death: The American Tobacco Industry*, Ashland, OH: Beech Tree Books, 1988.
Wi-Cancer.info. "Antenna Sickness Is Everywhere Now," [Undated]. Retrieved 2018 from http://www.wi-cancer.info/antenna_sickness.aspx.
Winnick, Michael, and Robert Zolna. "Putting a Finger on Our Phone Obsession—Mobile touches: a study on humans and their tech," Dscout, June 16, 2016. Retrieved 2018 from https://blog.dscout.com/mobile-touches.
Wireless History Foundation. "Wireless History Timeline," [Undated]. Retrieved 2018 from http://www.wirelesshistoryfoundation.org/wireless-history-project/wireless-history-timeline.
World Health Organization. "Electromagnetic fields and public health: mobile phones," October 2014. Retrieved 2018 from http://www.who.int/mediacentre/factsheets/fs193/en/.
Wyland, Scott. "Put cellphone down while driving in Italy or risk losing license," *Stars and Stripes*, July 26, 2017. Retrieved 2018 from https://www.stripes.com/news/europe/put-cellphone-down-while-driving-in-italy-or-risk-losing-license-1.479858.
Zada, Gabriel, MD, et al. "Incidence Trends in the Anatomic Location of Primary Malignant Brain Tumors in the United States: 1992–2006," *World Neurosurgery*, March–April, 2012: Volume 77, issues 3-4, pages 518–524. Retrieved 2018 from https://doi.org/10.1016/j.wneu.2011.05.051.

About the Author

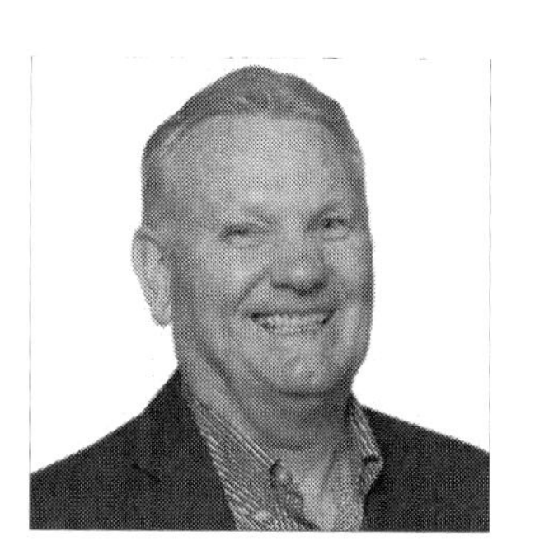

Bill Cadwallader is a Certified Electromagnetic Radiation Specialist, and one of 34 international EMF experts featured at the International EMF Health Summit. He has presented multiple times at the Annual Cancer Convention, multiple times at the Doctors Symposium in Los Angeles, and has taught at the Building Biology Institute. He serves as a coach for Building Biology Institute's Apprentice Program.

As a Certified Electromagnetic Radiation Specialist, Bill has completed advanced studies in electromagnetic radiation. Electromagnetic Radiation Specialists measure radiation and consult for detection and protection in homes, schools, and businesses. He detects and reduces all of the electromagnetic radiation threats to your home, family, children, environment, and even pets.

Bill has spent his adult life working around technology, from the time he joined the U.S. Marine Corps until he retired as a Lieutenant Colonel (Reserves), as a postgraduate student at Pepperdine University, and as a Project Manager in the Aerospace Industry in California, as well as working in the Information Technology Department for Clark County, Nevada.

Prior to consulting in electromagnetic radiation, he became concerned about the amount of radiation people were being exposed to in their daily lives. When a co-worker was diagnosed with brain cancer, Bill was shocked. He remembered that he always saw his co-worker on his cell phone, before meetings and after meetings. The brain tumor was located at the exact place where he held the cell phone to his head.

The man later died, after massive medical treatment. Bill knew something was very unsafe about the way people were using their cell phones and other electronic devices. After another acquaintance developed a tumor in his abdomen, right where he held his tablet every night to read, he knew he had to do something.

Now, as a Certified Electromagnetic Radiation Specialist, Bill provides on-site EMF Inspections in Nevada, Utah, Arizona, and Southern California. He also speaks extensively on solutions to harmful electromagnetic radiation. He can be reached at StopDirtyElectricity.com.

Bill holds a Bachelor of Science Degree from Cal Poly Pomona, Pomona, California, and a Master's Degree from Pepperdine University, Malibu, California.

Bill was born and raised in Bakersfield, California, and resides in Las Vegas, Nevada, with his wife, Lois.

877-783-6465

x 702-845-5794

Acknowledgements

I am eternally thankful for:

The GIANTS: Outspoken Experts, Pioneers and Colleagues:

Devra Davis, PhD, MPH; Magna Havis, PhD; David O. Carpenter, MD; Lennart Hardell, MD, PhD; Olle Johannson, PhD; Joel Moskowitz, PhD; Sam Milham, MD, MPH; Martin Graham, PhD; Cindy Sage, MA; Henry Lai, PhD; Lloyd Morgan, BS; George Carlo, PhD; Martin Blank, PhD; Martin Pall, PhD; Arthur Firstenberg, BA; Dietrich Klinghardt, MD, PhD; Louis Slesin, PhD; Andrew Marino, PhD, JP.

The following Certified Electromagnetic Radiation Specialists:

Larry Gust, Rob Metzinger, Spark Burmaster, Oram Miller, Diana Schultz, Nancy Messinger, Eric Windheim, Liz Menkes, Lee Sagula, Paul Doyon, and Frank Cousineau and Lorainne Rosenthal of Cancer Control Society.

Many thanks to Larry Gust, Electrical Engineer, BBEC, EMRS, for his technical review of this book. Mr. Gust has an electrical engineering degree and an MBA from the University of Wisconsin. He was a member of management at Dow Chemical and at Mobil Corporation from 1977 to 1992, working in manufacturing, product development and total quality management. Mr. Gust has been teaching classes and seminars for IBE since 1996. Since 1993, under the banner of Gust Environmental, he has been conducting residential and commercial building assessments and recommending remedial plans for indoor air quality and electromagnetic issues. Mr. Gust is the president of the IBE Board of Directors. He is an IBE certified Building-Biology Environmental Consultant and a certified Electromagnetic Radiation Specialist.

Special thanks to Oram Miller, BBEC, EMRS, my continuing education coach, who inspired me to go far beyond what my dreams used to be.

Family and Friends: To all who have who have perfected the many evolutions of my speaking presentations.

Suzanne Cadwallader, Janis Cadwallader, Lynn Cadwallader, Richard Barran, Arthur Raybold, Valerie Bennett.

Tim and Nancy Wezeman, Luke and Cara Wezeman, Emma Wezeman, Josh and Wendy Penner, and Don and Jamie Ely.

Phyllis Palmer, Marc and Micah Jordan, Heidi Harris, Brad and Karen Balon, Dale and Melody Butler, Robin Skone-Palmer, Jean Olson, Carolyn Clark, Susan Babajtis, Nancy Meserve, Jodymarie Cushman, Tim Baurley, Robert D. Milne, MD, and Dr. Robert Goodman, DC.

Kathi Minsky, the Internet master who conceived, designed, and oversaw construction of all things related to websites, social media, and Internet marketing.

Many thanks to SMH Design Solutions for all of its work on Design & Development, Web & Social Media Marketing, and Communications & Brand Strategy.

George Stamos, who gave me the sub-title for this book, the Electronic Sickening of America, and his wife, Charlene Stamos, for her valuable input and patient support.

Erica, Holly, and Erin Calkins, who lit the fire to complete this book.

Bert Decker and Dru Scott Decker, my communications mentors.

Special thanks to Farren Lander for his encouragement and resources that contributed to my speaking presentations.

Larry Edwards, editor and publishing consultant.

Lois Cadwallader, my loving wife and very best friend, who has encouraged me to be the best at anything I take on. Without her writing ability and her tenacity to investigate the research, this book would never have been completed and delivered.

All of the people who have families that need to know how to avoid the most catastrophic cancer and disease epidemic since tobacco was first rolled into cigarettes and gave me the inspiration for writing book.

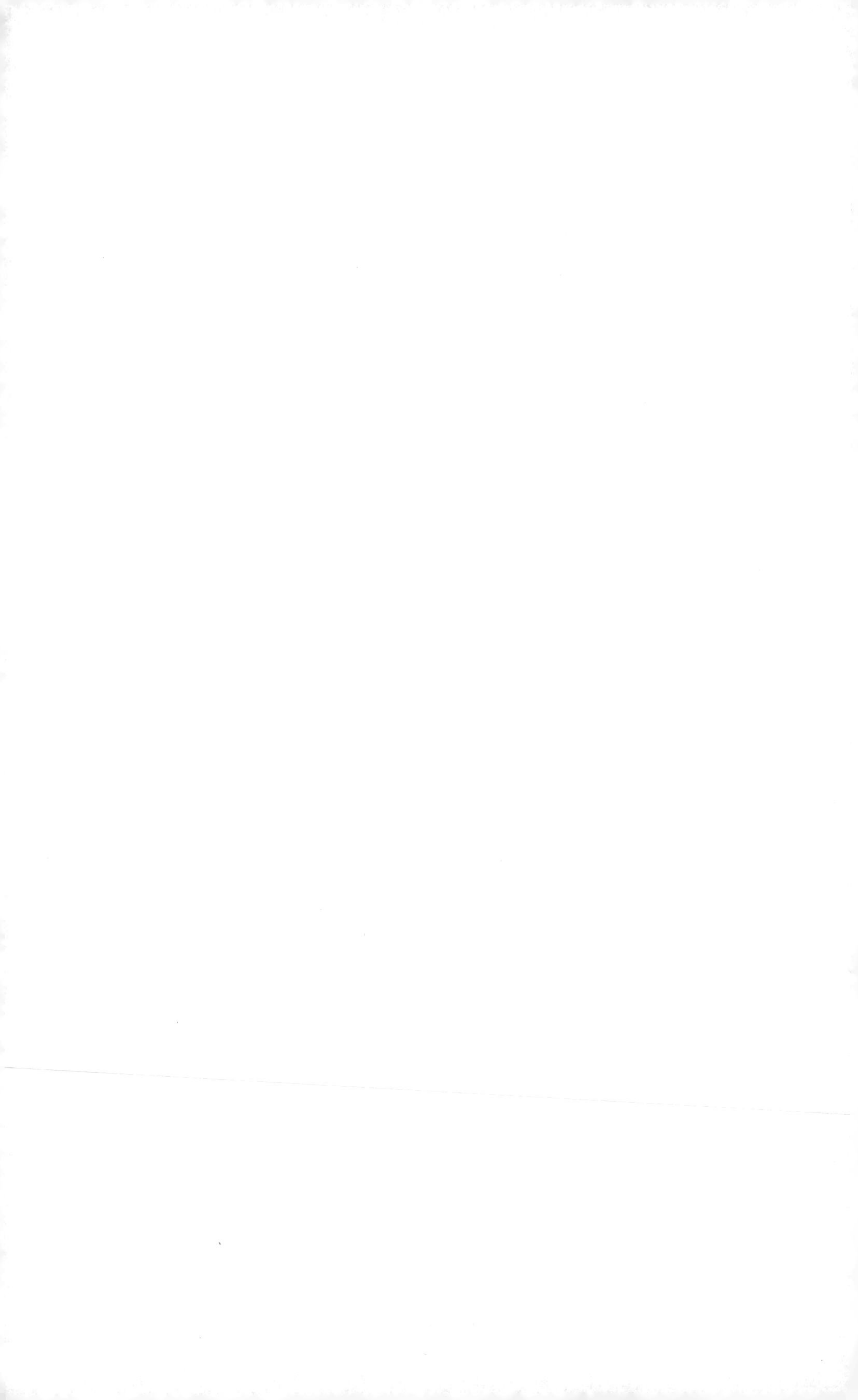

Made in the USA
Middletown, DE
14 January 2021